Bircher-Benner Manuals

Manual for patients with multiple sclerosis, Parkinson's disease and other neurodegenerative diseases

Dietary instructions
for their prevention and healing,
with recipes, detailed advice
and a treatment plan
from a medical centre
dedicated to state-of-the-art healing.

Dr. med. Andres Bircher
and colleagues of the
Bircher-Benner Medical Centre,
Lilli Bircher, Pascal Bircher and
Anne-Cécile Bircher.
Bircher-Benner Manuals

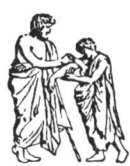

EDITION BIRCHER-BENNER
CH-8784 BRAUNWALD

Bircher-Benner Manuals

1. Manual for patients with multiple sclerosis, Parkinson's disease and other neurodegenerative diseases
2. Manual for patients with liver and gallbladder conditions
3. Manual for families and children
4. Manual of fresh juices, raw vegetables and fruit dishes
5. Manual for improvement of the immune system and against susceptibility to infection
6. Manual for mountaineers and athletes
7. Manual for diabetics
8. Manual for support and preventive therapy for lung diseases
9. Enjoy food without table salt
10. Manual for patients with rheumatism and arthritis
11. Manual for men with prostate conditions
12. Manual for patients with kidney and bladder conditions
13. Manual for venous diseases
14. Manual for patients with gastro-intestinal conditions
15. Manual for nutrition during pregnancy and lactation
16. Manual for gynaecological problems and menopause
17. Manual for the prevention of cancer and accompanying therapies
18. Manual for headache and migraine
19. Manual for patients with hypertension, cardiovascular disease and arteriosclerosis
20. Manual for overcoming anxiety and depression
21. Manual for patients with skin diseases or sensitive skin
22. Manual for persons suffering from stress
23. Manual for persons suffering from allergies
24. Manual for prevention of dementia and Alzheimer's disease
25. Manual for internal treatment of eye problems
26. Manual for treatment of weight problems, overweight, and anorexia

These manuals are the result of global research, the development of the art and science of medicine over more than a century, and the experience of the renowned Bircher-Benner Klinik. The reader will benefit from the helpful support of the well-informed physician every step of the way.

3rd edition fully revised, 2018. Translated from the original German.

All rights reserved, including the right of reproduction in excerpts, photomechanical reproduction and translation.
info@bircher-benner.com   www.bircher-benner.com

Book orders: edition@bircher-benner.com
© Copyright Edition Bircher-Benner, CH 8784 Braunwald
® The trademarks Bircher and Bircher-Benner are protected worldwide
Printed in Germany

The suggestions in this book have been carefully reviewed by the authors and the publisher. However, we cannot assume any guarantee. The authors and the publisher hereby disclaim all liability for personal injury, property damage and any type of financial loss.

Cover design: Kösel Media GmbH, Krugzell
Overall production: Kösel, Krugzell

Table of Contents

Preface 7

Introduction 9

The structure of the central nervous system 10
    The cerebrum 10
    The thalamic nucleus 11
    The cerebellum 12
    The limbic system 12
    The hormone-producing glands of the brain 13
    The anterior lobe of the hypophysis (adenohypophysis) 13
    The posterior pituitary (neurohypophysis) 14
    The epiphysis and melatonin 14

The nerve cell (neuron) 15

The potential for action 16

The synapses 17
    Messenger substances of the nervous system (neurotransmitters) 17

The importance of the glial cells in the brain 18

The spaces of the brain and the fluid in the brain and spinal cord 19

The blood-brain barrier 20

Transport through the blood-brain barrier 22

The behaviour of the blood-brain barrier in substance transport into
and out of the brain 23

The effect of alcohol consumption on the blood-brain barrier 24

The effect of smoking on the blood-brain barrier 25

The effect of electromagnetic radiation on the human brain
and the blood-brain barrier 26

The myelin marrow sheaths – a sensitive substance 27

Demyelinating diseases 28

Remyelination 29

Guillain-Barré syndrome (GBS) 30

Diseases from storage of degenerative proteins 31
    The TAU proteins 31

Amyloidosis 32

The effect of nutrition on the central nervous system 33
    Two kinds of food energy 33

The basic regulation system of the soft connective tissue
in the central nervous system 35

Oxidative stress at the centre of the causes of neurodegenerative
diseases 37

The influence of environmental stress from pollutants as the cause
of neurodegenerative diseases 39
    The neurotoxic effect of mercury 39
    Organic tin compounds and neurodegeneration 40
    Chlorine and neurodegenerative diseases 41
    The neurotoxic effect of volatile organic hydrocarbons 41
    Insecticides and neurodegenerative diseases 42
    Wood protection agents and neurodegenerative diseases 43
    Neurotoxic medicines and neurodegeneration 43

Legal and prohibited drugs and neurodegenerative diseases 44
    Cannabis 44
    Amphetamines 44
    LSD (lysergic acid diethylamide) 44
    Heroin, morphine, other opiates 45
    Nicotine 45

Alcohol	46
Caffeine	47
Regarding the phenomenon of primary and secondary effects and the danger of polypragmasia from medication	48
The combined effect of harmful neurotoxic substances	48
Vitamins, trace elements and neurodegenerative disease	49
The various types of neurodegenerative diseases	51
Systematic overview of neurodegenerative diseases	51
Multiple sclerosis	53
Causes of multiple sclerosis	55
Genetics	55
The infection hypothesis	55
Vitamin D and MS	56
Mercury exposure and multiple sclerosis	57
Scientific basics for nutritional therapy in multiple sclerosis	59
Progresses of multiple sclerosis	63
The symptoms of multiple sclerosis	64
Diagnosis of multiple sclerosis	65
Medical treatment of multiple sclerosis	66
Order therapy for multiple sclerosis	68
Supporting measures for nursing of the patient, water applications	71
Hydrotherapy for MS patients	71
Emptying the intestine	75
On the general lifestyle with multiple sclerosis	76
Parkinson's disease	78
The causes of Parkinson's disease	78
Nutrition and Parkinson's disease	80
The symptoms of Parkinson's disease	81

The mental effects of Parkinson's syndrome	82
Ensuring diagnosis of Parkinson's disease	82
Atypical Parkinson's syndrome	83
The treatment of Parkinson's disease	83
Comprehensive treatment for Parkinson's disease	85
Dietary treatment of neurodegenerative diseases	86
Lab control recommendations for the attending physician during the diet	89
Practical application of the raw food therapy	93
Menus	94
Menus for various raw food regimes	94
Daily menu	96
The Recipes	98
Juices	98
Bircher muesli	99
Fruit and fresh grain dishes	100
Chilled soups	101
Milk types	101
Raw vegetables and salads	102
Salad dressings	103
Suggestions for dressings to go with the salads and raw vegetables	106
Cooked food	107
Recipes for cooked food	107
Vegetables	110
Salads of cooked vegetables	114
Potato dishes	115
Cereal dishes	117
Sauces	119
Sandwiches	121
Recipes Index	123
Notes	125
Index	137

Preface

All neurodegenerative diseases cause horrendous suffering for the patients. Congenital forms are very rare. The most common diseases are multiple sclerosis, Parkinson's disease and Alzheimer's disease. Amyotrophic lateral sclerosis follows a particularly tragic course and is diagnosed with increasing frequency. There is no consensus as to the cause, but it is impossible not to link the steady increase of these diseases in all Western countries – whose typical nutrition features large quantities of animal protein and fat, white flour, sugar, coffee and alcohol – with sedentary lifestyles and insufficient sleep before midnight. Neurodegenerative diseases usually progress slowly, with degenerative inflammatory processes in various parts of the nervous system. The search for a pathogen (e.g. a virus) causing multiple sclerosis was long conducted in vain, until we understood that viral infections are not directly involved in the disease, but only act as a trigger by weakening the immune system.

In the last thirty years, many scientific works have uncovered an increasing number of partial causes of multiple sclerosis, such as excessive weight, lack of exercise, animal-based nutrition including a large quantity of meat and fatty cheese, lack of polyunsaturated vegetable oils, vitamin D deficiency, oxidative stress, stress from environmental toxins, the effects of industrially synthesised nutrition and an unnatural lifestyle.

The focus of scientific medical thinking is on the autoimmune processes, i.e. the destructive attacks of the immune system on the structures of the body's nervous system, the nerve cells and the sensitive myelin-containing nerve sheaths. This explains why all therapeutic efforts to combat multiple sclerosis are focused on medication designed to suppress pathogenic autoimmune inflammation. In some cases, this treatment can briefly delay the bouts of illness, but it can also have dangerous side effects. Immune suppression does not target the cause of the disease. The disease progresses continually in spite of an immense effort with pharmacological medication.

Only recently have the significant geographical, epidemiological differences in the frequency of multiple sclerosis been taken seriously. Attempts have been made to comprehend this, leading to the understanding that differences in nutrition and lifestyle, rather than genetics, are the cause. All of these data and scientific studies suggest strongly that the poor nutrition common in Western industrialised countries is the cause.

Lymph cells are formed in the bone marrow. They then migrate into the mucosa of the intestine, which is permeated with dense lymph cell nests, like a leopard's skin. Our intestinal milieu is complex. The closest continuous contact between the body's substances and external substances takes place there. In the lymph cell nests of the intestinal mucosa, immune cells (i.e. dentric cells) are continually "trained" to differentiate between the body's own substances and external substances, both beneficial and harmful, and to recognise pathogens. Only 10 % of the lymphocytes pass this test and will migrate into the lymph nodes and all tissues of the body as immuno-competent cells. A healthy intestinal mucosa is covered by a dense layer of mucous. This is infused with IgA-antibodies. The IgA-antibodies form a catalogue of what is compatible, according to prior experience, and thus not to be fought with an immune response. Autoimmune diseases, such as the autoimmune inflammation in multiple sclerosis, result when the intestinal milieu is impaired because of a degenerated intestinal flora that attacks the intestinal mucosa with putrefactive toxins. The result is that the mucous layer and its antibody catalogue are deficient. This causes the mucosa barrier – which separates the intestinal content from the inside of the body – to leak, and the immune system of the intestine will begin to react to a number of different foods. In multiple sclerosis, there is usually a large number of IgG4- and IgE-mediated food incompatibilities. Eating such foods damages the intestinal mucosa still more. An unhealthy intestinal milieu prevents the correct transformation of the cells of an enteral immune system into immuno-competent cells. The ability to distinguish between external and internal substances becomes imperfect, so that the immune system increasingly attacks body tissue and tends to produce autoimmune inflammations.

Many scientific studies indicate the importance of nutrition-related metabolic toxins and deficiencies that damage the myelin sheaths of the nerve cells and pathways. Other scientific works point out clear interrelations between multiple sclerosis and the effects of certain environmental toxins and heavy metals. Additionally, there is new damage to the central nervous system from today's all-pervasive stress on people, coming from pulsed high-frequency radiation from mobile phones, wireless house phones, WLAN and other wireless connections. The highly significant relevance of such harmful exposure to the human brain has been documented, even though it can be expected that this will only be accepted over time because of the powerful personal and outside interests of most politicians.

This book presents a comprehensive therapy that targets the causes of multiple sclerosis, Parkinson's disease and amyotrophic lateral sclerosis, to the extent to which these are known today. The causes and prevention of the various forms of dementia and Alzheimer's disease are treated in Bircher-Benner manual no. 24. This book is based on all the modern scientific insights that are relevant for the understanding, prevention and effective causative treatment of neurodegenerative diseases. Additionally, it must be added that multiple sclerosis has already been treated for more than a hundred years. Our greatest teachers are the many patients who have been successfully treated at the famous Bircher-Benner Klinik in Zürich and at our medical centre over the years with our vital vegan fresh food diet, new life order and the careful elimination of toxin stress, foci of diseases and interference fields. This book provides the patient and his family with practical instructions for successfully treating and arresting multiple sclerosis and for preventing Parkinson's disease and amyotrophic lateral sclerosis, or for positively influencing their courses once they have already developed. For the treating physician, this book is a great help for the instruction and guidance of his patients.

Introduction

To understand the causes of multiple sclerosis and other neurodegenerative diseases, to the extent to which that they are known today, it is important to have some basic knowledge regarding the construction and function of the central nervous system. In fact, multiple sclerosis may attack and damage the central nervous system anywhere. Therefore its forms are very diverse. Parkinson's disease has a much more consistent course, since it is always caused by an attack on and degeneration of the nucleus niger, a pigmented core in the corpus striatum, one of the basal ganglia of the brain. Amyotrophic lateral sclerosis also follows a typical course, since it almost exclusively affects the motoric nerve pathways that are responsible for muscle strength and action and therefore causes increasing paralysis.

The explanations concerning some of the anatomical and functional situations in the central nervous system help to reveal the causes of these diseases and enable every patient to actively contribute in preventing and healing multiple sclerosis. This is a very rewarding undertaking.

The structure of the central nervous system

Estimates suggest that the human brain is made up of nearly 100 billion nerve cells (neurons). The number of glial cells (i.e. the cells that protect and feed the nerve cells that keep the living conditions of the neurons constant and that are part of the immune system of the brain) is similarly large.

The cerebrum

The largest number of nerve cells is located in the cerebrum, embedded in the connective-tissue-like supporting framework of the glial cells, in many windings (gyri) and furrows (sulci). The cerebrum is divided into the frontal lobes, the temporal lobes and the occipital cortex. There is a deep furrow on either side (sulcus centralis). The frontal parts of the cerebrum in front of this furrow mostly serve action-related purposes (executive cortex), while those behind it are assigned to sensitivity, perception and sensation. The foremost part of the frontal lobe (prefrontal cortex) contains the key structure for a circuit that controls decisions and considers whether a decision should be taken in view of potential benefits and disadvantages. The other convolutions of the brain in the frontal lobe (lobus frontalis) are important for personality development, for clearly focused thinking and for problem-solving skills[1].

The convolution directly in front of the central furrow contains the nerve cells for all movements, like an inverted "little man" or homunculus (homunculus, motor cortex), with a particularly large number of neurons assigned to the tongue, the hands and feet. If these were stimulated, the body would respond by moving the respective limb on the other side of the body. If the nerve cells in the next convolution in front of it were stimulated, the body would respond with more complex spontaneous movements. If nerve cells in the temporal lobe were stimulated, the body would respond with complex spontaneous movements.

Behind the central furrow, there are nerve cells that receive sensations from all body regions (sensory cortex). The left temporal lobe contains cell formations that permit speech (Broca's area). The frontal lobes are important for focused, targeted thinking and decision-making, and for guiding and controlling emotions and urges. The occipital cortex contains the centre of visual perception through the eyes (visual cortex).

There are two long protrusions at the front beneath the frontal lobe. This is the olfactory bulb, which is directly connected to olfactory cells. The nerve cells of the cerebral cortex are grey (grey matter). The nerve fibres (neurites) leading away from them consist of white matter.

This matter is white because its nerve fibres are surrounded by lipid-containing (fatty) marrow sheathes that appear white. They protect the nerve fibres (axons) and provide much faster conduction of nerve impulses. The two halves of the cerebrum are linked closely to each other by white nerve fibres. This connection is called the corpus callosum.

Below this on both sides is a very primal part of the brain, which is reminiscent of a sea horse in shape (hippocampus). The hippocampus is where information from different sensation-processing systems (sensory systems) is brought together, processed and returned to the cerebral cortex. The hippocampus is very important for strengthening the memory (i.e. for transferring contents from short-term memory to long-term memory), thereby producing the capacity of memory. After severe emotional trauma, such as war or the consequences of sexual abuse, the hippocampus may shrink (atrophy). However, it has been proven that the neurons in the hippocampus are able to regenerate given the right conditions.

The basal ganglia
Deep inside, between the hemispheres of the cerebrum, are the basal ganglia. They are considered to be part of the cerebrum. Part of them, the 'striped' core (corpus striatum), is divided into the pale core (globus pallidus) and a longitudinal core with a head and a tail (caudate nucleus). The large pathways from the cerebral cortex to the spinal cord run between these. The corpus striatum is a large switchboard that takes in information from the cerebral cortex and controls it by inhibition, like a coachman controlling his horse, and passes it on to the black core (nucleus niger), which in turn controls movements and coordination by inhibition and passes on its information to the thalamus.

The thalamic nucleus

The thalamic nucleus is the 'gate to the conscious mind'. All information emanating from the cells and the specialised sensory cells of the body, the cerebrum and the basal ganglia, are routed towards it. The thalamus selects the information supplied to the conscious mind and therefore forwarded to the cerebrum. The thalamus does not work autonomously, but rather is subject to the strict control of the cerebrum. Therefore we speak of the corticothalamic system in the context of the development of consciousness. The visual and auditory pathways from the eye and the inner ear are also connected via the thalamus, except for the olfactory bulb, which has pathways that go straight to the cerebral cortex. The corticothalamic system regulates the sleeping-waking rhythm and the general activity level of the cerebrum, as well as the vegetative nervous system, and controls general protective reflexes such as breathing, swallowing, sneezing and coughing.

The colour of the black matter (substantia nigra or nucleus niger) is the result of this core containing a large quantity of iron and melanin pigment. It has been carefully studied since Parkinson's disease results from the neural degeneration of this ganglion. The nerve fibres run from it to the cerebral cortex and the corpus striatum. Outbound nerve fibres go to the thalamus. The melanin-containing nerve cells (neurons) of the nucleus niger produce a significant quantity of dopamine and thus regulate the entire circuit of motion control. In Parkinson's disease, these cells degenerate so that the inhibiting control mediated by dopamine grows weaker and weaker. This produces the symptoms of Parkinson's disease: marked trembling (tremor), rigid facial expression, slower movements and gait, and stiff muscles, all described in detail in other chapters in this manual.

In addition to the inhibiting control of the black nucleus, the motoric movements are also controlled through inhibition by nerve cells from two other basal ganglia: the pale core (globus pallidus) and a core below the thalamus. When these fail, the control of the black core (nucleus niger) becomes predominant, which leads to the continuous, tormenting, excessive spontaneous waving movements of Huntington's disease, a congenital disease, or chorea minor if these cores are affected in the scope of the autoimmune reactions of rheumatic fever.

The black core can be viewed as one rein of the coachman, and the globus pallidus with the subthalamic nucleus as the other. If one rein is pulled too strongly, the motion disorder of Parkinson's disease results; when the other one is pulled too strongly, choreatic disorder results.

The cerebellum

The cerebellum is located on either side below the occipital lobes. Its primary function is to coordinate movement and walking. The cerebellum and the "bridge" (pons) are collectively called the hindbrain (metencephalon). The pons is a bulge of nerve fibres between the midbrain (mesencephalon) and the afterbrain (myelencephalon).

The brain stem, the medulla oblongata and the spinal cord

The pons and the myelencephalon form the brain stem, from which the medulla oblongata leads down to the spinal cord. The pons is a passage for all pathways that interconnect the "upstream" and "downstream" areas of the central nervous system, such as various cerebrum areas to the spinal cord (tractus corticospinalis). The pons contains collections of nerve cell (nuclei pontis) that connect the cerebrum to the cerebellum during decussation. The medulla oblongata contains nerve cell collections (nuclei) that control the vital functions, respiration and the heart (respiratory, cardiac and blood pressure centres).

The limbic system

The structures of the limbic system form a double ring around the basal ganglia and the thalamus. The limbic system is formed partly by phylogenetically old sections of the cerebral cortex (archipallium) and brain structures that are placed below the cerebral cortex. The name comes from limbus (seam), since the system is situated as a ring below the cerebrum hemispheres on both sides. This includes the hippocampus, fornix, corpus mamillare, gyrus cinguli, corpora amygdalae, front parts of the thalamus, septum pellucidum and a brain convolution at the side of the hippocampus.

To the limbic system is ascribed the processing of emotions and it is linked to all the other brain structures.

Damage to the limbic system produces the following neuropsychological defects: inability to assess emotional situations, memory problems, post-traumatic stress disorders, autism, depression, phobias and narcolepsy (inadvertant sleeping during the day). Alzheimer's disease damages the hippocampus (part of the limbic system) at an early stage, so that emotional disorders occur early on. Schizophrenia will often reveal reduced circulation in the limbic system in PET scans. Bipolar disorder is also ascribed to damage to the limbic system. Neuroleptics and sleeping pills, such as benzodiazepines (Valium, Temesta, etc.), have a manipulatary effect on the limbic system. In neurodegenerative diseases, degenerative damage to the limbic system is largely responsible for personality change.

The nerve pathways for moving the body's muscles (tractus corticospinalis) cross at the level of the medulla oblongata, so that any stimulation of a left side motoneuron of the left cerebral cortex leads to a reaction in the right half of the body. The cerebral cortex contains the "first" motoneuron (proximal motoneuron). Its long nerve extension (neurite) reaches down into the spinal cord in long pathways until it contacts a segment assigned to it (level). There the nerve extension (neurite) reaches its assigned second nerve cell (distal or second motoneuron) in the foremost lateral part (anterior horn), which may have a very long nerve pathway to the assigned muscles.

The same course in the reverse direction is taken by sensory nerves (sensitive nerves and nerve pathways). Their first nerve cell is located in the organ or skin area that produces the sensation. Their nerve extension (neurite) reaches into the posterior horn of the spinal cord in the segment (spinal cord level) assigned to it, where it passes on its perception to a second nerve cell (second neuron). The nerve fibres of all of these second neurons run as rear strands in the rear spinal cord up to the thalamus, where they are switched and selected (as previously described) before transmitting the information to the cerebral cortex and into the conscious mind.

The hormone-producing glands of the brain

The best-known of the hormone-producing glands is the pituitary gland (hypophysis). The hypothalamus is located below the thalamic nucleus. It controls the hormone production in the body by measuring the hormone concentrations in the blood and adjusting them to the current demand. If the amount of specific hormone to be produced is to be increased, the hypothalamus will send a substance (hormone-releasing factor) to the pituitary gland, which will cause the corresponding hormone to be produced to an increasing degree.

The anterior lobe of the hypophysis (adenohypophysis)

The following hormones are produced:

Thyroxin releasing hormone (TSH)
This stimulates the thyroid cells to increase production of thyroid hormones T3 and T4. If their levels (concentrations) in the blood grow too high, the hypothalamus will register the fact and reduce its stimulation again.

ACTH (adrenocorticotropic hormone)
Its excretion is regulated in the same manner. It stimulates the glandular cells of the adrenal glands to increase the production of cortisol.

FSH (follicle stimulating hormone)
This is regulated in the same manner and stimulates the production of oestrogens and the follicle maturation of the ovum, as well as the production of sperm in the male.

LH (luteinising hormone)
Causes ovulation and stimulates the production of progesterone (gestagen) for the production of the corpus luteum. In the male, it stimulates production of the masculinising hormone testosterone, which is also relevant in the female but in a lesser concentration.

PRL (prolactine)
This stimulates the mammary gland to produce milk while at the same time inhibiting the production of sex hormones (gonadotropins).

STH or GH (somatotropin or growth hormone)
This promotes body growth as long as the epiphyseal plates remain open. It promotes the release of fatty tissue and conversion of fat into sugar. It releases the insulin-like growth factor (insulin-like growth factor IgF1).

MSH (melanocyte-stimulating hormone or melanotropin)
It stimulates the pigment-forming cells (melanocytes) to increase pigment production.

The posterior pituitary (neurohypophysis)

Its two hormones are formed in the hypothalamic nucleus and these migrate down into the posterior pituitary, which in turn releases them into the blood. These two hormones are:

ADH (adiuretin or vasopressin)
This hormone causes the integration of resorption channels (aquaporin) into the collective tubes of the kidneys, so that more water from the primary urine is absorbed back into the blood.

Oxytocin
This hormone causes the uterus to contract and milk to be excreted by the mammary glands.

The epiphysis and melatonin

The epiphysis is about 7 mm large and located at the very rear, below the corpus callosum. It produces the hormone melatonin when it becomes dark outside. Synthetic light suppresses its production also, and this impairs sleep. It has been documented that melatonin is very important for learning and spatial memory[2]. Melatonin plays an important role in regulating the circadian rhythm and sleep. In the United States today melatonin is sold over the counter as a sleeping pill. However, the National Institute of Aging has issued warnings about the casual use of melatonin.

The nerve cell (neuron)

Each of the approx. 100 billion nerve cells of the brain comprises a cell body with cytoplasm and a nucleus. One or several protrusions grow from this to receive the information (neurites), along with a very long protrusion that forwards the information (neurite). The protrusion can be more than one metre long. All of these protrusions contain cellular fluid deep inside, as well as mitochondria for cell respiration and a supply of energy-providing phosphates. The nerve cell and dendrites belong to the grey matter of the brain, since they have no myelin sheaths that would colour them white.

The dendrites
Dendrites have multiple branches and are able to find other nerve cells and nerve fibres with their endings, thereby amplifying the linking of information in the central nervous system. This adjustment is very important in the development of the brain in children and is retained to an advanced age. The learning of new skills, thinking, cognitive tasks and making music all promote new links. If skills are not needed, the links between the dendrites are removed. This adaptability is called brain plasticity.

The neurites
Neurites are the forwarding nerve fibres. They run through the brain and spinal cord in bundles and pathways and combine in the body into nerve roots and nerves. The inside of the neurites is called the axon (Greek for axis). It contains the cell membranes, cytoplasm and mitochondria, and is fed from the cell body. The axon is enveloped by cells of the connective tissue of the brain (glial cells), by multiple convolutions of a myelin-containing layer, 95 % of which are made of fats, with a high content of cholesterol and polyunsaturated fatty acids that colour the neurites white. The body nerves have special cells (Schwann cells) that produce the myelin sheaths. The myelin sheath is constricted after a little less than every thousandth millimetre (nodes of Ranvier). Stimulation jumps from node to node. This increases the nerve conduction speed considerably.

The potential for action

Potassium is pumped in and sodium out at the membranes of the nerve cells, thereby producing an electrical potential of about 80 thousandth of a volt (mV, resting potential) at the cell membrane. When the nerve cell receives a large quantity of information from its dendrites, the potential increases until there is a discharge, and the nerve cell transmits information through its neurites.

If the nervous system is overstimulated, the resting potential increases and little is required to produce a discharge. If the resting potential is reduced, the nerve cell will react late and slowly. A high magnesium level and a high calcium level in the blood stabilise the nervous system, while low sodium or high potassium considerably increases its excitability.

The synapses

These are connections in which signals are transferred by one nerve cell to another or to muscle fibres. The complexity of the dendritic networking in the brain is extremely differentiated. A cerebellum cell, for example, will take up signals from other cells through about 100,000 dendritic synapses. Transfer of the action potential via the synapses usually takes place through chemical transmitters (neurotransmitters).

There are different types of synapses: those with stimulating and those with inhibiting messenger substances.

Messenger substances of the nervous system (neurotransmitters)

Stimulating messenger substances

Glutamate is the most important exciting neurotransmitter of the brain and is involved in many processes, such as the controlling circuits of motor control in the basal ganglia, where Parkinson's disease and Huntington's disease result. A special glutamate receptor, the NMDA receptor, is involved in learning processes[3].

Noradrenaline is located in many synapses of nuclei of the brainstem. In the vegetative nervous system of the body, it transfers the signals of the ganglia (control centres) of the sympathetic nervous system (stimulating vegetative system).

Adrenaline is not a neurotransmitter, by contrast. It is excreted only as a hormone by the adrenal gland and unfolds its effect at the synapses of noradrenaline throughout the organism.

Acetylcholine acts on the parasympathetic (calming) vegetative nervous system in the ganglia and at the synapses of the transfer of signals of the motoric nerves to the muscle fibres (motoric end plate).

Inhibiting messenger substances in the brain

GABA (γ-aminobutyric acid) is the most important inhibiting messenger substance of the brain. GABA acts at the synapses of many nuclei in the brain. Members of the group of medicines of the benzodiazepines (Valium, Temesta, etc.) act at the GABA receptors of these synapses and cause a general dampening of the central nervous system in this way. They have a sedative effect, and thus reduce anxiety and muscle tension.

Glycine is an inhibiting neurotransmitter that is mostly found in the spinal cord.

Serotonin plays a role especially in the area of the brain stem and the pituitary gland. It has a certain mood-lifting effect. Depression can be alleviated by adjusting the serotonin level through medication.

The importance of the glial cells in the brain

The name 'glia' comes from Greek and means 'glue'. The supporting function of the glia cells and their fibres for the nerve cells (neurons) were recognised at an early stage. Most glial cells come from the outer layer of the germ layer (ectoderm), but the microglial cells are from the middle layer (mesoderm). As far as we know today, the glial cells not only form a supporting structure for the nerve cells, but they also provide electrical insulation with their protective envelopes. Furthermore, the glial cells are involved essentially with substance transport and fluid exchange, and in maintenance of the homeostasis in the brain. Additionally, they contribute to the process of information processing, storage and forwarding. Glial cells are usually smaller than nerve cells. In the posterior pituitary (neurohypophysis), specialised glial cells (pituicytes) influence transport, storage and release of the hormones adiuretin (ADH) and oxytocin by the nerve fibres.

Most glial cells of the brain are astrocytes that resemble stars with their many protrusions. They regulate the potassium and fluid balance in the brain and the acid-base balance. They are also involved in processing of information in the brain. They contain vesicles with the stimulating neurotransmitter glutamate. Its release can activate adjacent nerve cells. If nerve fibres (axons) are injured, they form glial scars. However, this prevents new growth of the nerve fibres and thus prevents healing of paraplegia. Special astrocytes function as important conductive structures in the early development of the brain. The oligodendroglia cells form the myelin for the electrical insulation of the nerve fibres (axons).

Microglial cells make up about 20 % of all glial cells. During brain development, they ensure the correct number of predecessor cells for the nerve cells (neurons). Then they participate in immune defence by turning into macrophages. Since antibodies cannot enter the brain across the blood-brain barrier, the microglial cells are responsible for the immune defence against inflammation in the brain. They also support the nerve cells in regeneration after injury[4]. Thus the microglial cells have a function similar to that of macrophages in the immune system in other tissues, since they remove the cell residues of dead nerve cells and oligodendrocytes by phagocytosis (absorption and dissolution).

It is assumed that the microglial cells are produced from predecessor cells of the blood-forming system just like the other immune cells in embryonic development. They also act as antigen-presenting cells in the brain once they are activated by a suspicious molecule. This activation is, for example, involved in the degenerative inflammation processes of multiple sclerosis. Like amoebae, they migrate to the site of the inflammation and gather there. Once they arrive there, they remove cell toxins such as hydrogen superoxide or nitrogen monoxide from dead cell substances and foreign bodies. After breaking down defective body tissue and foreign substances, they emit specific cytokines (interleukin-1, tumour necrosis factor α, interferon γ) into the space outside of the cells (extracellular space). In this way, the astrocytes reduce and form glial scar tissue.

The spaces of the brain and the fluid in the brain and spinal cord

The fluid in the brain (liquor cerebrospinalis) is excreted from the two lateral cavities (lateral ventricles) made up of capillaries, a type of vasoganglions (plexus chorioideus). This ensures substance transport from the blood to the brain in a highly complex manner and at the same time prevents unacceptable substances from getting from the blood to the meninges and the brain fluid (blood-brain barrier). From the lateral ventricles, the brain fluid flows into the middle third ventricle, from there into the fourth ventricle below, and from there into the thin spinal canal at the centre of the spinal cord. The brain fluid then enters the space of the web-like cerebral membrane (meningea arachnoidea) and is resorbed into the blood. The brain fluid contains only little protein in a healthy person and very few white blood corpuscles.

The blood-brain barrier

The blood-brain barrier protects the brain from pathogens, toxins and messenger substances circulating in the blood. It is a highly selective filter through which the nutrients needed by the brain are supplied, and metabolites produced in the metabolism are discharged. This entire substance exchange is ensured by a great many ingeniously conceived transport processes.

The blood-brain barrier is only very rarely the cause of disease, but is very often stressed by it. It usually holds back medicines, so that the pharmaceutical industry has to carry out significant research to bring medicines to the desired place to affect the brain. The blood capillaries are very carefully sealed from the brain tissue by 'tight junctions'. Glial cells keep careful watch over the capillaries being sealed.

The brain's mass makes up only 2 % of the body's total mass. Its share in the nutrient demand is approx. 20 %, however. In contrast to the other bodies, the brain has almost no nutrient and oxygen reserves. Nerve cells can survive for no more than three minutes without oxygen. The brain cannot handle interferences with the acid-base balance (pH-deviations). Fluctuations of the potassium content must not reach the brain any more than should the messenger substances of the synapses (neurotransmitters) that circulate in the blood vessels. The great impermeability of the blood-brain barrier to pathogens, antibodies and white blood corpuscles (leukocytes) circulating in the blood makes them an immunological barrier so that the cells of the microglia must take over the function of the immune defence.

The high energy demand of the brain produces an above-average amount of metabolites that must be discharged through the blood-brain barrier.

The complex functions of the brain are bound to highly sensitive electrochemical and biochemical processes that can only run in a constant inner environment, homeostasis, usually without interference. Changes to the blood-brain barrier cause changes to the condition of the central nervous system, which in turn may cause function impairment or diseases of the central nervous system. Accordingly, a number of neurological diseases are connected to changes to the blood-brain barrier.

The brain is permeated by more than 100 billion capillaries, the total length of which has been calculated to be approx. 600 km[5]. The cerebral cortex contains 300 to 800 capillary cross sections per mm^2. The total area of the blood vessels in the brain is estimated at 12 to 20 m^2 [6,7], making the sealing of this large area of capillaries extremely difficult. The cells that form the capillary walls (endothelial cells) are thin.

In contrast to the capillaries in the remaining part of the body, they are sealed by being attached to each other (tight junctions). The astrocytes of the macroglia monitor the formation and sealing of the endothelial cells and place complex end feet on the capillary walls for sealing purposes.

Highly specialised cells of the microglia (pericytes) regulate cell division of the endothelial cells in the capillary walls. They secrete the substance actin, with which they change the diameter of the capillaries and thus regulate the blood pressure in the brain vessels. These pericytes are also able to convert to macrophages, eliminate foreign and toxic substances, and present antigens to the immune cells[8, 9, 10, 11].

Transport through the blood-brain barrier

The membranes of the blood-brain barrier contain fat (lipophilic). Nevertheless, tiny molecules (less than 0.52 nm^2) can diffuse through the blood-brain barrier. This is made possible by a very small kink of a membrane molecule producing a tiny gap that goes through the membrane with the molecule[12, 13, 14]. Fat-soluble (lipophilic) substances generally pass most easily through the plasma membranes of cells made of fatty acids. Nevertheless, in patients six years old and older, 98 % of the medicines that are of small, fat-soluble molecules and etheric oils are no longer able to enter the brain.

Small molecules with a polar charge, such as the water molecule, can only diffuse through the wall of the capillaries within very strict limits through the hydrophobic kinks. Nevertheless, large amounts of water can pass the blood-brain barrier to the brain. For this purpose the membranes contain hydrophilic (water-soluble) protein molecules (aquaporins, canal proteins). Glycerine and urea molecules can also pass through such canal proteins.

There is a special transport system for the transport of glucose and amino acids to the brain in the capillary membrane (GLUT-1 transporter). Other transport systems (MCT-1 and 2) can transport organic acids, such as lactic acid, pyruvic acid (pyruvate), mevalonate, butyrates and acetate. There are special transport systems for nutrients, vitamins, hormones, trace elements and folic acid as well.

There are very special transport systems for various larger molecules that consume energy. Selected large molecules, such as the iron-containing transferrin or the LDL cholesterol, which is very important for the brain, are fed through the membrane of the capillaries by small vesicles (vesicular transport) and include insulin and other peptide hormones and cytokines for immune defence. Other selected peptides (short-chained proteins) and proteins (larger protein molecules) are fed through the membrane because of their positive charge (cationic transport)[15].

Many neurodegenerative diseases, but also diabetes, considerably impair the blood-brain barrier. Certain pathogens can pass this barrier as well, including the HI and other viruses and bacteria, such as Neisseria meningitidis or the cholera bacterium (Vibrio cholerae)[16].

The behaviour of the blood-brain barrier in substance transport into and out of the brain

Extremely fat-soluble, unpolar substances (solvents) and chlorated hydrocarbons pass unhindered through the lipid-containing membranes of the blood-brain barrier into the brain. Other substances, such as many nutrients (amino acids, sugar, vitamins) can only pass the blood-brain barrier using active and passive transport systems. All of the cell types named for the blood-brain barrier form a functional system that is also called a 'neurovascular unit'. This ensures unhindered transport of vital nutrients from the blood, removal of the degradation products of the metabolism from the brain into the blood, and the recognition and elimination of harmful foreign substances or toxins if these are not fat-soluble. The blood-brain barrier has specific substance transport systems for this purpose.

Larger molecule complexes, viruses and small particles are transported in small vesicles that are fed through the membrane in a complex manner. Some of these transport systems are only active in one direction. One is the P-glycoprotein system in the membrane of the capillary walls. This binds foreign and hazardous substances to its receptor (PgP receptor) and foreign and hazardous substances from the brain into the blood. The blood-brain barrier can also feed neurologically and immunologically active substances such as nitrous oxide (NO), prostaglandins and cytokines (messenger substances from immune cells) out of the brain into the blood.

On the other hand, the blood-brain barrier is less tight in the liquor cavities (brain ventricles) and the olfactory brain, so that activating messenger substances (cytokines such as the interleukins IL1-α, IL1-β, IL-6, TNF-α and interferon IFN-γ) from inflammations and suppurative foci of the body, the intestine or from abscesses of tooth roots can enter the brain from the body. These activate the immune system of the microglia and are therefore largely responsible for the chronic inflammatory processes in the brain that cause multiple sclerosis and the other neurodegenerative diseases[17].

Various studies also showed that 12 different interleukins can cross the blood-brain barrier and thus get from the blood into the brain. It has been documented that various cytokines, including IL1-α, IL1-β, TNF-α and IFN-γ, can enter the brain if they are highly concentrated in the blood. This has led to the conclusion that there must be specific transport systems for these cytokines in the membrane of the endothelial cells of the capillaries of the brain[18].

The effect of alcohol consumption on the blood-brain barrier

Alcohol consumption damages the blood-brain barrier. It is a main risk factor for inflammatory diseases of the nervous system and for susceptibility towards bacterial infections[19, 20, 21]. Damage to the blood-brain barrier from alcohol is considered to be an essential influence for the development of some neurodegenerative diseases[22]. Damage to the blood-brain barrier is documented by neuropathological examinations of alcoholics as well as in animal experiments[23]. In the animal experiment, it has been found that the enzyme myosin light-chain kinase (MLCK) that is activated by alcohol consumption causes phosphorylation of several tight junctions or cytoskeletal proteins in the endotheliums, where the integrity of the blood-brain barrier is impaired[24]. Alcohol consumption leads to significant oxidative stress that additionally damages the blood-brain barrier[25]. It is not the alcohol as such, but its degradation products (metabolites) that activate the myosin light-chain enzyme (MLCK) in the endothelial cells of the capillary walls. The damage to the blood-brain barrier from consumption of alcohol assists the ingression of white blood corpuscles (leucocytes) into the brain, which facilitates inflammatory processes in the brain such as the ones relevant for multiple sclerosis[22].

The effect of smoking on the blood-brain barrier

It has been shown in several studies that smokers have a much higher risk of developing dementia from Alzheimer's disease than non-smokers[26]. Extended administration of nicotine to test animals changed the function and structure of the blood-brain barrier[27]. In epidemiological studies, a much higher risk of bacterial meningitis has been documented for smokers[28].

The effect of electromagnetic radiation on the human brain and the blood-brain barrier

The harmful effect of the pulsed high-frequency radiation from mobile phones, in the mega- to gigahertz range, have been scientifically documented[29]. This applies similarly to the radiation from mobile house phones, wireless connections on computers, WLAN and remote controls. There is no consensus yet about the harm caused by the same radiation in a lower energy range. High energy density of electromagnetic radiation has been shown to cause considerable heating in the affected body tissue. In the skull, this heat can impair the blood-brain barrier and make it more permeable[30]. The power required for a 15-minute call by mobile phone heats the brain much less than a hot bath, though heating from the bath causes no damage[27]. The Swedish university in Lund proved that the blood-brain barrier, as well as the neurons of the brain, can be damaged even without the effect of heating from a mobile phone's radiation[31, 32, 33, 34].

Physics differentiates between electromagnetic waves and scalar waves. Scalar waves are also used in mobile phones. They can pass through concrete walls like jackhammers and reach even a distant child's bedroom, the iron-reinforced basement in houses and the underground floors of supermarkets and other shopping centres. Physics differentiates between transverse waves (Hertz) and scalar waves (Tesla). Transverse waves cannot enter metal grids or cages (Faraday cage). They can hardly pass through reinforced concrete walls and ceilings, and cannot enter cars or elevators at all. One hundred years ago, Tesla discovered a wave type that cannot be held back by anything and that passes through everything: the scalar wave. This longitudinal wave is aligned lengthwise and forms wave vortexes. Today's mobile phones work mainly with scalar waves. Tesla made his first attempts with a personally constructed transmission station on a mountain meadow. A herd of cows was grazing there. His video shows that the cows turned wildly in circles every time he switched on the transmitter. When he switched the transmitter off, they went back to eating calmly.

The risk of damage is that our biological system works with scalar waves as well, e.g. the morphogenetic fields that affect the differentiation of body forms on the basis of the genetic material. Sunlight reaches us as a transverse wave and is converted into scalar waves (standing light wave equals photon) when entering the biological system. The sunlight is greatly amplified according to the LASER principle and saved in the genetic substance of the cells. The frequency pattern of the spontaneous brain activity in the electroencephalogram corresponds to that of sunlight. The human brain works with scalar waves; brain currents are disastrously cycled within the scalar wave frequency window of mobile phones at 10 Hz[35].

The myelin marrow sheaths – a sensitive substance

Myelin is a biomembrane that spirally envelops the nerve strands (axons). It is made of up to 70 % fats (lipids) and 30 % protein. Because of the high fat content, the fast-conducting nerve pathways appear white and consequently form the white substance in the brain. The fast-conducting nerve fibres in the body are also enveloped by myelin sheaths.

In the brain, myelin is formed by the cells of the microglia (oligodendrocytes); in the nerves in the body, myelin is formed by Schwann cells. Myelin is complex in its structure: myelin fats are 25 % cholesterol, 20 % galactocerebroside, 5 % galacto-sulfatide and 50 % mainly phosphatidylethanolamine and lecithin. The proteins are basic myeloproteins (MBP), proteolipid protein (PLP/DM20), myelin-associated glycoprotein (MAG) and connexin (CX32). In addition, myelin oligodendrocyte glycoprotein (MOG) appears in the brain, and protein zero (P0, MPZ) and peripheral myeloprotein-22 (PMP-22) are found in the nerves of the body. Proteolipid protein (PLP), also called lipophilin, is important for stabilisation of the marrow sheaths.

Congenital diseases with defective myelin formation, called leukodystrophies, are rare.

Demyelinating diseases

Demyelinating diseases occur because of damage to the myelin sheaths which eventually destroys the nerve fibre running at their centre. They can also be described as "de-marrowing" diseases.

Multiple sclerosis is by far the most common of these diseases. Other rare diseases are acute disseminated encephalomyelitis (ADEM), acute motoric axonal neuropathy, balo disease, chronically inflammatory demyelinating polyneuropathy, funicular myelosis, Miller-Fisher syndrome, transverse myelitis and Neuromyelitis optica (Devic's syndrome).

Remyelination

The oligodendrocytes of the microglia of the brain are able to repair the myelin sheaths. This regeneration capacity is extremely effective in the healthy brain. The repaired myelin sheaths are much thinner. With multiple sclerosis, however, remyelination is strongly impaired because of autoimmune processes, so that it is insufficient for healing.

At present, many research centres are seeking to understand why remyelination is not successful in multiple sclerosis. Apparently the stem cells of the oligodendrocytes do not mature. Messenger substances from inflammation cells (cytokines) inhibit maturation of the oligodendrocytes from their preliminary stages. The tumour necrosis factors 2 and α play key roles in this[36]. Chemokines conduct the oligodendrocytes to the place of degenerated myelin and promote maturing of the oligodendrocytes. In multiple sclerosis, chemokine CXCL12 is strongly reduced. Residues of degenerated myelin also are supposed to activate the cell receptor LINGO1, which prevents remyelination and maturation of oligodendrocytes[32]. With increasing age, remyelination declines. It is presumed that the genes responsible for this are reduced in their activity[37]. Certain growth factors promote remyelination, such as the factor EGF and others[32]. Certain cell receptors (toll-like receptors) have also been found that inhibit maturation of the oligodendrocytes and thus remyelination[38].

Many other factors and influences are being researched. In multiple sclerosis, it has been documented that remyelination initially is still very efficient, but fails as the disease progresses chronically[39]. Researchers are trying to find medicines to block the receptors Notch-1, Wnt and LINGO1, which inhibit cell maturation.

Guillain-Barré syndrome (GBS)

In Guillain-Barré syndrome, the myelin sheaths of the nerves responsible for motor control (motoneurons) of the body are attacked by autoimmune processes. This causes progressive paralysis, partially limp and partially spastic. The front nerve roots coming from the spinal cord (polyradikulitis) and the associated front nerve roots suffer the worst form of demyelination. The precise cause has not been determined. In two-thirds of the patients, an infection was the catalyst. Frequently documented pathogens include: Campylobacter jejuni, Epstein-Barr virus, cytomegalovirus and varicella zoster virus. These infections often leave behind a temporary weakening of the immune system. Guillain-Barré syndrome can also occur after flu or tetanus vaccination[40, 41].

Guillain-Barré syndrome may lead to paralysis rising up from the feet within hours, or much more slowly, over the course of months. When the paralysis reaches the respiratory muscles, the patient requires artificial respiration under intensive care. In 80 % of all cases, the paralysis disappears again entirely. However, every fifth patient will suffer permanent paralysis. Every year, two to three of every 100,000 people contract Guillain-Barré syndrome; men are affected slightly more frequently than women. Although rare, the nerves of the brain or sensory nerves may be affected as well and arrhythmia may occur when vegetative nerve fibres are affected.

Whether the paralysis is persistent or not depends on whether the organism manages remyelination before the naked nerve fibres (axons) are destroyed. Forms that attack these quickly and severely are called axonal forms. This includes acute motoric and sensitivity axonal neuropathy (AMSAN), which is more common in China and Japan, and acute motoric axonal neuropathy (AMAN). In North America, Guillain-Barré syndrome is diagnosed with the axonal forms with the worse prognosis in 5–10 % of the cases. A particularly slowly developing version is called subacute inflammatory demyelinating polyradiculoneuropathy (SIDP)[42].

If diagnosed early, Guillain-Barré syndrome can usually be healed completely. In acute and severe cases, immunoglobulin infusions and plasmapheresis are used[36].

Diseases from storage of degenerative proteins

The TAU proteins

The name is derived from the Greek letter TAU.
These are structural proteins that have been changed in their molecule structure by phosphorylation so that their task of being integrated in the microtubules of the cell skeleton can no longer be met. They are therefore stored in the nerve cells (neurons) of the brain, where they form twisted fibres (twisted fibrils). Nine of such diseases, called tauopathies, have been so far identified. The fibrils destroy the neurons entirely, resulting in a slow death to the brain.

By far the best known of the tauopathies is Alzheimer's disease. It also presents intense depositing of beta amyloids in the inter-cell substance, the basic substance of the brain. Alzheimer's disease is not a genetic disease. Causative connections have been documented in relation to widespread poor nutrition with too many animal products, to various environmental pollutants and to pulsed high-frequency radiation from mobile phones. The tauopathies, such as Alzheimer's disease, are treated in Bircher-Benner manual no. 24, on the prevention of dementia and Alzheimer's disease.

Amyloidosis

Amyloidosis means enrichment of abnormally changed proteins in the inter-cell substances, the basic substance of the soft connective tissue that runs through the entire body and ensures all exchanges of substances between the blood capillaries and the cells. The degenerative change renders the proteins insoluble in water. They are therefore present in the form of small fibres, called fibrils. They are called β-fibrils. These pathological deposits are caused by a pathologically changed metabolism resulting from widespread poor nutrition. The name of amyloid was given because these deposits look similar to starch under the microscope.

Amyloidosis is based on an interference in the folding of a usually soluble protein[43]. Many years of poor nutrition and several diseases may cause amyloidosis through impaired metabolism ecology, i.e. overproduction, missing or reduced breaking down or impaired excretion of certain proteins. The proteins are in a dissolved form in the blood vessels and capillaries. If their concentration increases, they will get into the inter-cell substance of the surrounding tissues and are attacked by enzymes. The combination of the resulting amino acid chains in the area of the β folding sheet structures forms insoluble complexes in the form of microscopically small fibres (fibrils). These fibrils are resistant to being absorbed by and into macrophages (phagocytosis and proteolysis by macrophages), and therefore can no longer be broken down.

In primary amyloidoses, there is no underlying disease to be found. These are rare and sometimes occur repeatedly in one family. Secondary amyloidoses are by far the most common ones. There is an underlying disease as the cause, such as chronic inflammation, chronic infection, tumours of the lymphatic system or long dialysis treatment.

Many elderly persons suffer from old-age amyloidosis, deposits in particular in the heart or brain, in the form of β-amyloid in the inter-cell substance, as is the case in Alzheimer's disease. This is also called AS-amyloidosis, or senile amyloidosis. The cause lies in widespread poor nutrition and the resulting considerable impairment of the metabolism. Amyloid deposits cause all kinds of function impairment in the brain and nerves, leading up to Alzheimer's dementia. There often are painful sensory or movement impairment in the nerves of the body (the peripheral nerves). If the vegetative nervous system is affected, the blood pressure will fall while the patient is standing (orthostatic weakness), there will be an early feeling of saturation due to reduced emptying of the stomach, erectile problems, impaired intestinal peristaltic with flatulence, stomach ache and irregular passing of stool. This book treats only the effects of amyloidosis on the central and peripheral nervous systems.

The effect of nutrition on the central nervous system

Two kinds of food energy

Physicists are aware of two types of energy: the orderly and the chaotic. Orderly energy saves information. Chaotic energy cannot save anything. Heat energy is chaotic energy. Sunlight is the most highly ordered form of energy. Its information is in a way similar to a large symphony. Listening to a symphony does not produce heat, but it provides information: it is a highly orderly sound structure that triggers precise sensations and feelings. With its complex oscillations, sunlight conveys and orders the genetically specified information that is needed for the growth, differentiation and regeneration of all life on earth.

One green leaf contains about one million chlorophyll funnels. At the base of each funnel, there are two chlorophyll α molecules each. The funnel reflects the incoming light into the base, where the chlorophyll A-molecules enter into a maximum resonance, synchronised with the oscillations of the solar radiation (coherence). They convert the energy from this resonance into UV light, which makes them light up (invisibly to our eyes). This light flows through the entire plant body, all the way to the roots and the tips of the roots[44, 45]. All living cells store UV light in their molecules, especially in the ring-shaped molecules.

The double helix of the genetic material in the cell cores stores by far the most light. The double helix (DNA) can coil to the right or left and can form protrusions shaped like clover leaves, radiating specific UV light spectrums[46]. The double helix of the DNA serves as a cavity resonator for the rhythmic LASER amplification of UV-light in our cells[47]. For a LASER to begin to work, it must receive a certain amount of energy. Bio-physicians call this minimum energy supply the LASER threshold. In their experiments, researchers of the International Academy for Biophoton Research measured the LASER threshold in plant tissues[43].

Just like plants, human and animal cells store UV-light in their DNA[48, 40]. We lack the ability to photosynthesise, however, and direct application of sunlight to the skin is far from enough to keep our LASER light storage above the LASER threshold.

The plant's cell stores the photons from sunlight in incredible intensity. It could be shown that the ultra-weak cell radiation[41] is nothing but a leakage radiation, a tiny leak of the UV-light through the cell membrane. Measurements showed that LASER amplification of the light is 10^4 times stronger in the DNA than that provided by technical LASER devices. Enzymes are activated 10^{10} times more strongly by light than by heat. The inside of the cells thus represents an incredible light space.

Our photon storage must be fed daily with a sufficient amount of vital photon-containing foods, i.e. fresh vegetable foods[49, 50, 51]. The transmission of the information of the vital foods from photosynthesis to our organism takes place by coherence. This means that our own sensation of life, life energy and life information is renewed and reordered again and again in the roughly 50 trillion cells of our body by entering into a shared resonance with the oscillation patterns of sunlight on the transfer of the photons (coherence).

If fresh, raw foods are missing from our nutrition, the photon content in our cells will decline. The light content will fall until it drops below the LASER threshold. The cells partially revert from the principle of order (coherence principle of Prigogine[52]) to the chaos principle of thermodynamics and degenerate.

We consider disease a loss of order, a loss of ordered information. The programme of life enters into disorder and the lack of fresh, raw nutrition makes reordering impossible. Numerous experiments which were conducted among others at the University of Novosibirsk[53] show that the complex processes of biochemistry in our cells are controlled by information. If there is a lack of fresh, raw nutrition, this information will no longer be continually renewed and ordered. Thus the complex biochemical processes of our cells will be thrown into disarray. This is why fresh, raw plant food is important for its energy: it renews and strengthens the ordering resonance.

The basic regulation system of the soft connective tissue in the central nervous system

All cells of the body's organs are embedded in the basic substance of the soft connective tissue that runs through all organs and structures. They are made up of a molecular network (matrix) of sugar-protein molecules called proteoglycans. The blood capillaries run through the basic substance, including the nerve endings of the vegetative nervous system. Outside of the central nervous system, the capillaries leak deliberately. This permits nutrients and hormones to leave them freely. They reach the cells through the network of proteoglycans, which serves as a molecular screen and information conduction system. We have seen that autoimmune processes of an unhealthy milieu in the intestine and a degenerated intestinal flora are stimulated because the immune cells are only able to acquire a defective immune competence under such conditions. The defective immune competence does not enable them to distinguish between external and internal correctly.

The situation in the brain is very different from that in the body. The capillary loops, which are particularly tight here since an especially large amount of oxygen and food is necessary, are sealed by the blood-brain barrier, as explained above. The neurons need an entirely different milieu than do the body cells, a milieu that is regulated and kept constant by the glial cells, particularly the astrocytes and the complex system of the transport cannels of the blood-brain barrier. We have seen that, on the one hand, the oligodendroglial cells of the connective-tissue-like microglia protect and envelop the nerve fibres, the axons, and that, on the other hand, they take over the development and function of the immune system in the brain by converting into antigen-presenting cells and macrophages that move through the matrix of the brain like amoeba to remove intruding germs and toxins. We have also seen that the oligodendroglial cells of the microglia can repair injury to the myelin sheaths, but that this ability to regenerate the myelin, the marrow sheaths of the quick-conducting nerve fibres, is exhausted in multiple sclerosis due to the long-term autoimmune inflammation.

We have seen that abnormal degenerated proteins (amyloids) are deposited in the matrix of the brain tissue if the metabolic economy is not ensured and that these deposits of β-amyloids in the basic system of the connective tissue of the brain are one of the central causes of dementia from Alzheimer's disease. We have also seen how certain proteins that are supposed to help stabilise the cell membranes (cytoskeleton) change abnormally under the same prerequisites, making them phosphorylated. Instead of accomplishing their tasks, they become twisted fibrils that destroy the nerve cells of the brain.

Food economy and food energy play a key role in keeping the matrix and the basic regulation system with the network of proteoglycans beyond the blood-brain barrier healthy, both in the body and in the central nervous system. We will see below that the depositing of toxic heavy metals, oxidative stress from an unnatural lifestyle, poor nutrition and electromagnetic radiation damage not only the proper function of the blood-brain barrier, but also the basic regulation system of the brain and the neurons themselves, as well as the myelin sheaths, directly and severely, so that the immune system of the brain spins out of control and attacks the damaged degenerating tissue and the myelin sheaths through an autoimmune reaction that destroys the marrow sheaths and thus causes multiple sclerosis. The key to understanding the causes of multiple sclerosis and other neurodegenerative diseases is to be found here. It is the key to a treatment that is particularly effective for this disease and that is described in this book.

Oxidative stress at the centre of the causes of neurodegenerative diseases

Unsuitable nutrition, irritants, environmental stress, a disorderly lifestyle, ionising, and electromagnetic and UVA radiation all cause the organism to suffer from oxidative stress. This results in a metabolic situation in which in the physiological context a totally excessive amount of reactive oxygen compounds (R.O.S., or reactive oxygen species) occurs. These highly reactive oxidising substances are molecules with at least one unsaturated electron pair, which makes them particularly reactive. They are produced in the mitochondria, the 'power plants' of the cells that break down glucose through electron transfer and the enzyme Cytochrome P 450-oxidase. This produces the super oxide anion radical O_2-hydrogen peroxide (H_2O_2) and the hydroxide radical (OH) or nitroxygen (NO).

Healthy cells can neutralise these highly reactive oxygen compounds with neutralising substances that they keep ready for this purpose. The most important antioxidative substance provided by the body is glutathione, a peptide that it produces from the three amino acids glutamic acid, cysteine and glycine. Other important antioxidants are ubiquinone (of coenzyme Q10), vitamins A, C and E, selenium and many secondary plant substances from vegetable food.

In the case of oxidative stress in the metabolism, these reserves will have been depleted, and oxidised glutathione can then no longer be returned to its active, reduced form sufficiently, since the enzyme glutathione reductase is depleted, as well as other detoxification enzymes such as peroxide dismutase and catalase. The highly reactive oxidants (R.O.S.) thus remain in the metabolism, where they can damage large molecules (macro molecules) inside and outside the cells. This has dangerous consequences. The unsaturated fatty acids of the cell membranes are oxidised (lipid peroxidation), and this causes the destruction of the mitochondria, the power plants in the cells, exhausting the cells and requiring them to expend much more energy in order to maintain their electrical membrane potentials. Additionally, the lipid-containing myelin sheaths of the fast-conducting nerve fibres in the brain and the spinal cord and in the nerves outside of the central nervous system are damaged by lipid peroxidation. Additionally, there will be further damage to proteins (protein peroxidation) and the hereditary material (DNA peroxidation), which causes the DNA molecules of the hereditary material to split (genetic mutations) and may lead to the conversion of healthy cells into tumour or cancer cells. This is a premature ageing process, which significantly impairs life expectancy[54, 55, 56].

Glucose metabolism (in the respiratory chain of the mitochondria) produces water as its end product. In about 2 % of the cases errors occur so that, for example, an oxygen atom will connect to one instead of two hydrogen atoms. This will always create a highly reactive fission product of water: the hydroxide radical (OH*). This free radical is very reactive since the oxygen atom of the OH* radical is actively searching for an additional electron from another molecule. Other radicals include nitrous oxide (NO*), the chloride radical (Cl*), the bromide radical (Br*).

The importance of the free radicals is currently the object of much scientific interest in connection with research into the causes of various neurodegenerative diseases, such as Alzheimer's disease (AD), multiple sclerosis (MS), amyotrophic lateral sclerosis (ALS), Huntington's disease and Parkinson's disease. Many studies suggest the destruction of the brain stem ganglions by free radicals as a cause of these increasingly common diseases. Multiple sclerosis shows indications of damage to the myelin sheaths from free radicals, so that the immune system reacts against the oxidised lipids. The same happens in diabetic neuropathy[57].

It is accepted among scientists today[58] that oxidative stress holds a key position among the causes of neurodegenerative diseases. The process starts with the oxidation of proteins and enzymes, which change their spatial structure (tertiary structure) because of their oxidation and form an insoluble beta folding sheet structure that is then deposited in the brain in the form of aggregates – LEWY bodies in Parkinson's disease and β-amyloid plaques in Alzheimer's disease – where they destroy the nerve cells.

Usually, the correct folding of the protein is achieved by using special protein complexes (chaperones). It is suspected that these chaperone complexes are changed by oxidative and nitrosative stress, so that they can no longer perform their function in the production of a correct three-dimensional structure of the proteins. The insoluble degenerative proteins deposited inside and outside the nerve cells cause programmed cell death (apoptosis). Cell death is caused by excessive excretion of the activating neurotransmitter glutamate. Glutamate activates a receptor in the cell membranes (NMDA receptor) that trips a permanent calcium flow into the nerve cells. This activates an enzyme (NO-synthase), which causes the nitrous oxide radical (NO) to form. In the mitochondria, excess calcium inhibits cell respiration. This causes massive formation of free radicals (R.O.S.). The radical NO is oxidised further into the highly reactive peroxynitrite. Together with the other free radicals (R.O.S.), it damages the membranes immensely through lipid peroxidation. This releases the substance cytochrome C, which starts the biologically determined cascade of cell destruction (apoptosis).

The brain has a cell-preserving substance that protects the nerve cells from destruction by apoptosis. In this way, they would be protected from healthy adjacent cells. Since the adjacent cells are also attacked, this protection factor is missing and cell death spreads through the tissue of the brain.

The influence of environmental stress from pollutants as the cause of neurodegenerative diseases

Recent research has shown the direct toxic effects of many chemicals that in the brain lead to neurodegenerative diseases in the long term. For example, even low concentrations of mould as well as chemicals in the domestic environment may cause behavioural and memory problems[59]. This effect involves the glial cells, which are immunologically active, form part of the blood-brain barrier and are in direct, close contact with the nerve fibres.

The neurotoxic effect of mercury

This metal, which is a liquid at room temperature, is one of the most toxic chemical elements on our planet. Nevertheless, it has been introduced into the teeth of many millions of people in the last 160 years in the form of amalgam fillings. It is available as a salt in mono- and bivalent forms (Hg^+, Hg^{++}). Organic mercury compounds are formed from this as well, in particular the highly toxic methylmercury ($CH_3^- Hg^+$). Tooth amalgams contain more than 50 % mercury, as well as silver, copper and tin; these metals too are neurotoxic. In 2006, approx. 2000 tons of pure mercury were processed into tooth amalgams and used in dental fillings[60]. It is characteristic of the mercury in amalgam fillings that it evaporates constantly, so that concentrations of up to 52 µg/m³ air have been measured in the mouth[61]. The amount of evaporation depends on the number of amalgam fillings and the pressure exerted when chewing[62]. In the brains of people with amalgam fillings, concentrations of mercury two to twelve times higher have been measured than those in the amalgam-free control group[63]. Amalgam is transferred from the mother to the unborn child. Several studies showed that the mercury content in the brains of infants who died of sudden infant death correlated with the number of amalgam fillings of the mothers[64].

This meets the toxicological criterion of the dosage effect principle. Under the microscope, the highly toxic effect of mercury on the nerves can be observed and filmed directly. Even a concentration of 0.1 µMol/litre results in rapid degeneration of the nerve fibre (axon). A concentration of 0.18 µg Hg leads to a deposit of β-amyloid and a protein hyperphosphorylation by binding phosphorus to the TAU-protein, both of which are present in Alzheimer's disease[65]. This shows the extreme neurotoxicity of even very small doses of mercury – much lower concentrations than those measured in the organs of amalgam carriers. Additionally, these tests only used the ionised mercury Hg^{++}, rather than the much more toxic elementary mercury gas Hg, which passes the blood-brain barrier unhindered.

The gaseous mercury is ionised in the cells to become Hg^{++}. It then connects to the hydrogen sulphide groups of the proteins of organic substances such as hormones, neurotransmitters, peptides and enzymes. The mercury also inhibits the transport of calcium, sodium and potassium in the cell membranes, since it blocks their transport systems.

Additionally, mercury salts in the organism connect to methyl groups ($Hg-CH_3$).

Methylated mercury is fat-soluble. Therefore, it collects in the myelin sheaths of the brain, the spinal cord and the nerve sheaths. This impairs functions of the brain and spinal cord and leads to signs of peripheral polyneuropathy (nerve damage) such as trembling, impaired sensation and paralysis. Additionally, methylmercury causes the release of free radicals (R.O.S.) in the mitochondria of all cells. Through increasing oxidative and nitrosative stress, this causes nerve cells to die (apoptosis).

Mercury impairs the immune system severely and causes the release of cytokines (cell messenger substances) that trigger chronic inflammatory processes and provoke allergies. Mercury causes autoimmune diseases[66] and damages the dopaminergic D2-receptors of the basal ganglia of the brain, which in turn causes the symptoms of Parkinson's disease. Mercury also causes allergic diseases of the IV-type, such as hives (urticaria) and generalised eczema (neurodermatitis). In children, the appearance of a fully developed form of Feer's disease (acrodynia, Pink disease) also occurs, demonstrating all the symptoms of an allergic reaction to mercury together with marked psychical and dermatological symptoms in the children. Hair analysis best reflects the mercury deposits in the body tissues. Even mercury concentrations of 10–20 µg/g in the hair and 50 µg mercury/litre in the blood will cause mental and motoric retardation (development disorder of the brain).

Mercury is suspected of causing autism. The mercury stress of the mother (amalgams) during pregnancy is decisive in this. A mercury content of 10 µg/g hair is deemed a risk factor for development disorders of the brain in children[67]. Methylmercury may cause developmental disorders even in the embryo[68].

Alzheimer's dementia has increased considerably in Western industrialised countries since 1970. There are significant indications of connections between the poisoning of individuals with mercury and the increase in Alzheimer's disease[69, 70].

Organic tin compounds and neurodegeneration

Organically bound tin has an antibiotic effect. Therefore, it is used to refine textiles to reduce the smell of sweat that is caused by bacterial degradation. In particular it is applied to all sports textiles. In 2000, Greenpeace purchased sports jerseys from almost all the main sports goods producers and had them examined for their content of organic tin compounds. The PVC prints of the jerseys contained up to 10.2 mg organic tin compounds per kg fabric. These were monobutyltin, dibutyltin and tributyltin.

Organic tin compounds dissolve in fat so that they can enter the brain through the blood-brain barrier unhindered. Like lead, they block cell respiration in the mitochondria of all cells. The more carbon residues are bound to a tin atom, the higher their toxicity. Triphenyltin, trimethyltin and tributyltin may cause severe poisoning even merely on skin contact[71]. Tributyltin is one of the most dangerous and toxic substances that has ever been synthetically produced and spread in the environment, according to a joint press release of the WHO and Greenpeace in 2003. Tin poisoning results in symptoms of hyperactivity, insomnia, lack of appetite, and, later in life, general cramps. and mental confusion.

Trimethyltin may cause destruction of nerve cells of the brain through apoptosis. Trimethyltin causes an oedema (collection of water) in the brain and the spinal cord. This was shown in France in 1956 in a mass poisoning caused by an antiseptic (disinfectant) called 'Salinon' that killed more than 100 persons[72]. Tributyltin does not degrade well. In the animal experiment, it caused sustained chronic damage to the liver and bile ducts and to the immune system, with acute and chronic inflammation of the pancreas (pancreatitis) cancer and malformations (teratogenic effect) and hormone-like effects on the sexual organs and the sexual characteristics, even at very low doses[73].

Organic tin compounds release the interleukins IL-1α, IL-6, TNF-α in the brain. This leads to inflammation and degeneration, which attacks the hippocampus in particular. The hippocampus is decisive for memory and learning[74].

In humans suffering from organic tin poisoning, the nerve, glial and endothelial cells are unprotected from other chemicals, so that patients will suffer from intolerance to many chemical odors and vapours in addition to the toxic effect of the tin (multiple chemical sensitivity, MCS).

Organic tin compounds were used in the coats of paint on ship hulls to prevent algae and mussels attaching to them. They are so toxic that they have caused the mass death of fish, crustaceans and mussels. These paints were finally prohibited in 2003.

Chlorine and neurodegenerative diseases

Gaseous chlorine is highly toxic to the brain and nervous system. Nevertheless, it is still sold freely in cleaning agents and disinfectants for households in any number of drug stores. Javelle water is an aqueous solution of potassium or sodium chlorite. It has a strongly oxidising and corrosive effect. Javelle water should no longer be used at all. It is neurotoxic[75].

It is suspected that this is due to the hypochlorites, such as they are also used in swimming pools, which break down into elementary chlorine, hydrogen chloride, chlorine dioxide and oxygen even if heated only slightly.

The elementary chlorine gas that gives the swimming pool and cleaning agents their typical smell penetrates the blood-brain barrier unhindered and develops its neurotoxic effect in the brain. The following neurological symptoms indicate this: general oversensitivity to any chemical and its fumes, (multiple chemical sensitivity, or MCS syndrome), excessive pain in the arms and legs (hyperaesthesia and hyperpathia) with simultaneous reduced sensitivity to touch in the arms and legs, muscle weakness, reduced reflexes, melancholy and reduced mental and emotional resilience (Benton test). The ability to concentrate and to pay attention while under stress are especially affected.

These symptoms show that chlorine gas attacks the brain (toxic encephalopathy) as well as the peripheral nerves (polyneuropathy). From a neuropsychological point of view, this suggests a reduced 'working memory', the capacity for short-term information processing. This is caused by damage to the prefrontal cerebral cortex (frontal lobes) of the hippocampus, the limbic system and the brain stem. The positron-emission tomography (PET) showed reduced glucose turnover in parts of the cerebral cortex. Additionally, the affected patients often contracted cardiovascular diseases and Alzheimer's dementia at a young age and did not live beyond the age of 45 or 50[73].

The neurotoxic effect of volatile organic hydrocarbons

House painters, car painters and mechanics, carpenters and people who work in related industries are particularly exposed to paint components and solvents. It has been documented that even very small concentrations (in the microgram range) can cause neurotoxic damage over the years, which leads to a reduced ability to focus, fatigue and constant nausea[76, 77, 78]. Professional use of mixes of organic solvents causes severe neurotoxic damage at much lower concentrations[79].

It is important to note that the indicated MAK limits are politically negotiated values. Some of them are by a factor of 1000 greater than the scientifically determined references. In the hazardous substance mixtures, the individual references must be totalled in order to determine their toxicity[73].

Buildings treated with solvent-containing glazings and wood-protection agents may emit neurotoxic solvent vapours for a long time. If they produce disease symptoms (toxic encephalopathy), this is called 'Sick-Building Syndrome'[80]. The background stress on the population from vapours deriving from volatile organic solvents (VOC) is 300 µg/m³, while the effect threshold for chronic stress is much lower, at 200–300 µg/m³ [81]. Many widespread general complaints, such as fatigue, headache, sleeping disorders and lack of the ability to concentrate may have their cause in this background stress from solvent-containing paints and varnishes in rooms.

Insecticides and neurodegenerative diseases

Epidemiological studies have shown that the neurotoxicity of organic phosphorus pesticides is particularly relevant as the cause of chronic neurodegenerative diseases. Organophosphates were developed as chemical weapons by chemists of the arms industry in the early 20th century.

Today, they are marketed as insecticides for agriculture, under the names chlorpyrifos, thiodicarb, parathion, fenamiphos, azinphos-methyl and methamidophos. The toxic basic substance is an organic phosphoric acid ester.

These nerve toxins cause the following symptoms: oversensitivity of the skin to light, reddening of the skin, irritation of the eyes, acute problems with breathing, choking seizures (particularly in the evening), vertigo, paralysis of the arms and legs, rheumatism-like muscle pain (myalgia), growth impairment of the nails of the fingers and toes, tremor, hearing damage, vision problems, loss of coordination of movement (ataxia), nerve pain, lack of sensitivity in the legs (peripheral neuropathy), arrhythmia, damage to the memory (in particular in the short-term and working memory), anxiety, depression with the danger of suicide, change of personality with loss of emotion and urge control, and permanent irritation. These are slow, long-term effects that cause progressive loss of the will to live and the desire to maintain social relationships. The same high stress resulted in the Mosel region of Germany from eight treatments of the vineyards per year with organic phosphorus pesticides sprayed from helicopters and airplanes.

Progressive neurodegeneration grows worse for many years after the end of exposure to organic phosphorus pesticides, so that the personality continues to deteriorate. The PET topography of persons affected showed impairment in particular in the prefrontal lobe, which is important for weighing up advantages and disadvantages and for taking decisions; and in the gyrus frontalis inferior, which is important overall for the personality and moral behaviour, as well as for motivation coordination, short-term memory and problem-solving strategies. The visual cortex was also damaged (gyrus orbitalis). The relevant personality changes usually led to withdrawal and social isolation and to suicidal tendancies[82, 83].

The toxic group of molecules of organic phosphates blocks degradation of acetylcholine, causing this neurotransmitter to build up in the brain. Thus acetylcholine binds to stimulating muscarinic receptors, from where the glutamate receptors are stimulated, and this leads to general overexcitation in the central nervous system. Glutamic acid activates the N-methyl-D-aspartate receptor (NMDA), which is important for learning. However, this causes pathological inflammation. The muscarinic receptors occur in the frontal lobes, the hippocampus (important for memory capacity) and the basal ganglia. Excessive activation of these receptors further promotes the inflammatory processes. Permanent overstimulation of the NMDA receptor is deemed a primary cause of neurodegeneration through pesticides that destroys the mitochondria of all cells, lipid peroxidation of the cell membranes and myelin sheaths, and nerve cells by apoptosis.

Further neurotoxic harmful substances are used in daily life and at the workplace, as well as in family gardens: pesticides of the semi-synchronistic pyrethroid, type which are sold in any drug store and which providers recommend for use against vermin in the household and garden. They have a high neurotoxic potential.

Other neurotoxic heavy metals are found in batteries, accumulators, paints, jewellery, ceramic glazings, electronic devices and construction materials; these include cadmium, lead, thallium, nickel and chrome. They are often not disposed of as stipulated.

Other neurotoxic substances are found in flame retardants, such as polybromated diphenyl ether (PBDE) and tetrabrombisphenol A (TBBA). These substances are found in upholstery, electronic devices, carpets and cuddly toys for children. From there they slowly and continually enter the human organism and accumulate in the lipid-containing myelin sheaths of the brain. Since 1972, the content of toxic bromated flame retardants in breast milk has doubled every five years.

Wood protection agents and neurodegenerative diseases

Pentachlorophenol (PCP) has been prohibited since 1989, because it causes cancer and neurodegenerative diseases. In many old buildings, however, it is still present and emitting toxic vapours. Since the 1970s and 1980s, treatment of all prefabricated buildings containing PCP has been required. The neurotoxic effect of the newer replacement substances for PCP, among them dichlorfluanid, has not been sufficiently investigated. Hazardous long-term effects are quite possible.

Neurotoxic medicines and neurodegeneration

Prescription of neuroleptics of the family of the phenothiazine and butyrophenonedrugs in psychiatric clinics and practices is widespread. They cause the symptoms of Parkinson's disease by blocking the postsynaptic dopamine receptors and thus inhibiting the dopamine effect of the substantia nigra. Reserpine, as an isolated medicine or in Rauwolfia preparations, lowers the blood pressure and has a calming effect. It inhibits the presynaptic release of dopamine and may therefore trigger Parkinson symptoms.

Legal and prohibited drugs and neurodegenerative diseases

Cannabis

The active substances of cannabis, including tetrahydrocannabinol (THC), activate a dedicated group of receptors, mostly in the cerebral cortex. (CB 1 and CB 2). The nerve cells activated by this are connected to many others that, when affected by cannabis, release various neurotransmitters, such as acetylcholine, noradrenaline, dopamine, serotonin and glutamate.

As a *primary effect* of the drug, there is an increase in sensory impressions and sensations, changes in the perception of time, increases in feelings of well-being and self-esteem, relaxation and a reduction in the perception of pain. The *secondary effects (withdrawal effects)* are: hallucinations, anxiety, laughing fits, vertigo, impaired perception, delusions, paranoia and fatigue.

The neurotoxic long-term effects of cannabis are: memory and concentration disorders, motivation deficits, loss of drive, fatigue and idleness, increased risk of schizophrenia, psychotic episodes, brain damage and brain shrinkage (especially in the nucleus amygdalae).

Amphetamines

Amphetamines stimulate the release of monoamine neurotransmitters, such as serotonin, noradrenaline and dopamine. At the same time, they inhibit monoamine oxidase (MAO-inhibition), so that breakdown of excess neurotransmitters is delayed, especially in the area of the brain stem ganglia and the limbic system, where memory contents are linked to emotions.

The *primary effects* of methamphetamine, paramthoxiamphetamine (PMA) and other 'Ecstasy' drugs are: stimulation, improved physical performance, increased vigilance (awareness), reduced thirst and hunger, loss of inhibition, enhanced ego.

The *secondary effects (withdrawal effects)* are: sleeplessness, fear, depression, speech disorders, hallucinations, delusions, psychosis (schizophrenia), high blood pressure, high pulse rate. After large doses: cramps, respiratory arrest and kidney failure.

The *neurotoxic long-term effects* are: fatigue, sleeping disorders, emaciation, high blood pressure, paranoid hallucination, learning and memory disorders, a decline in intelligence, psychoses, dementia, degeneration of serotonin and dopamine-expressing nerves in the hippocampus and limbic system, increased risk of stroke and damage to the heart muscle (toxic myopathy).

LSD (lysergic acid diethylamide)

This drug has an activating effect on serotonin-(5-HT)-receptors in various brain areas, mostly in the brain stem, which are connected to the limbic system.

Primary effects of this drug are: hallucinations in colourful imaginary images, increased sensory perception, overstimulation.

The *secondary effects (withdrawal effects)* are: loss of control of the body and of thinking, impaired space-time perception, concentration and attention disorders, balance disorders, panic, delusions.

The *neurotoxic long-term effects* are: hallucinations and loss of a sense of reality. The potential for psychological addiction is moderate and that of physical addiction is low.

Heroin, morphine, other opiates

Opiates release endorphins.

Primary effect: euphoria (feelings of unnatural joy and excessive well-being), sedation (sleepiness), much reduced perception of pain, dullness, inhibition, enhanced ego, reduced perception (apathy towards others and oneself), reduced morality, respiratory arrest.

Secondary effects (withdrawal symptoms): lower blood pressure, slow pulse (bradycardia), fatigue, apathy, nausea, vertigo and considerable oversensitivity to pain in the body and limbs.

Neurotoxic long-term effect: depression, mood fluctuations, sleeping disorders, unstable moods, weak motivation, visual hallucinations, personality changes.

Nicotine

Nicotine also stimulates the acetylcholine receptors in the vegetative centres of the brain stem and the medulla oblongata, where the centres for blood pressure, respiration and the heart are situated. The ganglia of the sympathicus and parasympathicus (vagus) are stimulated at a lower dose and inhibited at a higher dose, until there is a receptor blockage. In the stimulation phase, neurotransmitters are released in various areas of the brain, among them dopamine, adrenaline, noradrenaline, acetylcholine, serotonin and β-endorphin. The blocking of these receptors is reflected in the secondary effect. High persistent doses of nicotine (chain smokers) will cause only the secondary and toxic symptoms.

Primary effect: cognitive performance, memory, attention, inhibition of fear, stress, pain, positive feelings.

Secondary effects (withdrawal symptoms): fast pulse, high blood pressure, nervousness, restlessness, impatience, sleeping disorder, irritability, inability to concentrate, reduced performance, reduced attention, sensitivity to pain, negative emotions.

Long-term neurotoxic effects: very strong physical and psychological addiction, discomfort, depression, toxic effects of heavy metals in cigarette smoke.

Other toxic effects: arteriosclerosis, cerebral sclerosis, heart attack, stroke, strongly increased cancer risk (benzoapyrene), emphysema of the lung.

Nicotine during pregnancy is neurotoxic for the unborn child. Smoking during pregnancy increases the risk of noticeable behavioural problems in later life that is 1.9 times as large; the risk is particularly high for ADHS syndrome (Attention Deficit Hyperactivity Syndrome). Exposure of the child to passive smoke after birth causes a 1.3 times increase in the risk of later behavioural disorders for the child. Smoking during pregnancy and passive smoke exposure after birth double this risk for the child.

Alcohol

Alcohol is fat-soluble and therefore penetrates the blood-brain barrier, so that the toxic effect on the nerve cells (neurons), glial cells and myelin sheaths is the main issue. Alcohol harms the blood-brain barrier directly and so severely that the brain becomes more susceptible to other toxins.

Primary effect: disinhibition, talkativeness, euphoric mood, reduced ability to think and make judgements, incapacity to control urges, sleepiness or aggressive behaviour, lack of emotional detachment, paralysis, speech and balance problems, blurred perception, loss of judgement ability, loss of consciousness leading to coma.

Secondary effects (withdrawal symptoms): vertigo, vomiting, headache, slower reactions, sleeping, balance and coordination problems, tremor, delirium tremens, paralysis, inability to think clearly, dulled thought processes, depression, irritatation.

Neurotoxic long-term effect: loss of mental capacity, reduced ability to make judgements, athylic dementia, personality changes, polyneuropathy with vitamin B_1 and zinc deficit (sensory impairment, pain), disrupted relationships, paranoia (paranoid ideas, paranoia persecutoria), destruction of personality, social decline.

Other toxic effects: severe liver damage, cirrhosis of the liver, pancreatitis and pancreatic cancer, increased risk of cardiovascular diseases, heart attack and stroke, chronic atrophic gastritis (stomach inflammation) with vitamin B_{12}-deficit, anaemia and degeneration of the sensitive pathways of the spinal cord.

Alcohol consumption during pregnancy
Analysis of several studies showed significant interrelations between the moderate alcohol consumption of the mother and development of ADHS syndrome in the child, starting with one glass of wine per week[84]. If the embryo (up to the 9th week of gestation) or the foetus (from the 10th week of gestation until birth) is exposed to alcohol or alcohol metabolites by the mother during development, such exposure will not simply impair development but may also cause severe physical and cerebral damage, depending on the stage of maturity. Alcohol enters the child's circulation unhindered so that the child is always subject to the same alcohol level as the mother during her consumption of alcohol. Thus even very low levels of alcohol during pregnancy will cause foetal alcohol syndrome (FAS) and alcohol embryopathy (AE), with significant mental disability and various physical malformations in the child. A minimal harmless level could not be found. After only one glass of beer or wine per week, emotional disorders and hyperactivity in children were already 37 % more common than in the children of the same age of abstinent mothers.

During the first three months of pregnancy, the most severe disabilities occur, in the forms of an abnormally small, malformed brain (microcephaly) and severe mental disability, malformations of the face and malformations of the body and internal organs. Alcohol consumption during the 4th to 6th months of gestation often leads to miscarriage. In the last trimester, the pregnancy is usually carried to term. Damage usually takes the form of a more or less severe mental disability, as well as severe delays in growth and development.

Foetal alcohol syndrome is the most common cause of mental disability without genetic cause[85]. In Germany, about 10,000 new-born babies every year suffer damage from alcohol. About 4,000 of them suffer from all the symptoms of foetal alcohol syndrome and will have severe mental and physical disabilities throughout their lives. The diagnosis is often not given in the case of less severe disabilities, so that an indefinite number of unreported cases must be expected. In a study of the Charité Berlin, 58 % of the pregnant women stated that they occasionally consumed alcohol[86].

Caffeine

The neurons (brain cells) have receptors for adenosine. When overstimulated and when their functions are overloaded, they produce adenosine, which binds to their receptors. This greatly reduces the reception of stimuli by the neurites, which is reflected in mental fatigue, slower thinking and inability to concentrate. Caffeine binds to the adenosine receptors of the neurons of the brain and displaces adenosine. This sabotages the protective natural blockage that normally allows the brain cells to recover and restores the ability to think and remain vigilant (wakefulness) for 1–2 hours.

Constantly repeated caffeine consumption in the form of coffee or 'energy drinks' contributes to chronic fatigue and degenerative changes in the neurons. Caffeine activates the stress hormone axis, so that adrenaline and cortisol are produced to a greater extent. This causes increased formation of cytokines and susceptibility to inflammation, also in the central nervous system.

Primary effect: restoration of vigilance (wakefulness) and clear thinking, brightening of mood, fast pulse, rise in blood pressure.

Secondary effects (withdrawal symptoms): increased fatigue, slower mental processes, sleepiness during the day, sleeping disorders at night, irritability, restlessness, insomnia, headache, overacidification of the stomach, impaired stomach and intestinal peristalsis. Reduced mental performance as a secondary effect after even just a single cup of coffee can be documented in psychological performance tests for up to one week after consumption.

Neurotoxic long-term effects: nervous mental exhaustion, headache and migraines. Bypassing the natural protective effect of the neurons leads to the expectation that caffeine might be a contributary cause for neurodegenerative diseases. This has yet to be examined scientifically.

Other toxic long-term effects of regular coffee consumption: migraine, headaches, high blood pressure, increased risk of cardiovascular diseases, heart attack, stroke, heartburn from reflux, stomach and duodenal ulcers, stomach cancer, increased risk of many cancer types from the carcinogenic contents of coffee (not from caffeine).

Regarding the phenomenon of primary and secondary effects and the danger of polypragmasia from medication

Primary effects are the first reaction to a medicine or a drug. After the relevant duration, which is specific to each drug, there will be a counter-regulation on the part of the organism that causes a secondary effect or reaction which is usually not desired. This phenomenon is generally not sufficiently taken into consideration when prescribing medicines, so that secondary effects are often viewed as a new symptom and further medicines are prescribed for them. The undesired side effects of medicines are typically secondary effects. When more than two drugs or medicines are taken, the interactions between the medicines can no longer be traced. Therefore the body's reaction cannot be predicted.

Undesired neurotoxic side effects of frequently prescribed medicines are common. They are very well recorded and described in medicine compendiums and files, as well as in packaging leaflets. To prevent neurodegenerative diseases, both the prescribing doctor and the patient must consider the undesired neurotoxic effects.

The combined effect of harmful neurotoxic substances

The effects of stresses from heavy metals, formaldehyde, dioxins, pesticides, solvents, drugs (including alcohol, nicotine and caffeine) accumulate so that compliance with the limits for individual substances when combined with others should be at a much lower level than what is acceptable for the individual substance alone.

Vitamins, trace elements and neurodegenerative disease

Vitamins A, C, E act as antioxidants in the metabolism. Vitamins A, D, E and K are fat-soluble. In the case of a massive overdose for an extended period of time, they may have a neurotoxic effect. A lack of vitamin B_6 and zinc prevents neurotransmitters from forming sufficiently.
A chronic pesticide stress will cause vitamin B_6 and zinc deficiencies.

A low blood level of the reduced form of folic acid (5 methyltetrahydrofolic acid) is associated with depression[87]. Where there is a vitamin-C deficiency, folic acid can only be converted into its reduced form (5-MTHF) in insufficient amounts. This reduced form (5-MTHF) is necessary, however, to convert homocysteine into methionine in combination with vitamin B_{12} in order to then form S-Adenosyl methionine. This is necessary for the formation of monoamine neurotransmitters. Additionally, reduced folic acid (5-MTHF) is needed for synthesis of adrenaline from noradrenaline in the adrenal gland.

A deficiency of folic acid causes the metabolism of the nervous system to become oversensitive to oxidative stress. This is indicated by an increased homocysteine level in the blood, which is due to a deficit of natural antioxidants, vitamin C, glutathione and NADH (nicotinamide adenine dinucleotide hydrogen). Accordingly, infusions with glutathione, vitamin C, folic acid and vitamin B_{12} have proven effective in treating persons with depression. A high homocysteine level, combined with a low concentration of B-vitamins (folic acid, vitamin B_{12}, vitamin B_6) is considered to be a risk factor for Alzheimer's disease and vascular dementia (dementia due to arteriosclerosis and vascular occlusion)[88]. Thus a high homocysteine level is regarded as a prognostic marker for the presence of a high risk of developing dementia. In 65-year-old patients, it can often be found together with a deficit in folic acid as well as in vitamins B_6 and B_{12}. This constellation is regarded as a preliminary stage of Alzheimer's disease. At the same time, it is an expression of oxidative stress from poor nutrition, an unnatural lifestyle, lack of sleep, chronic inflammation as in diabetes, then rheumatic inflammations, autoimmune inflammations and detrimental environmental influences (e.g. exposure of toxins and radiation), depression and Alzheimer's disease.

Vitamin D deficit is common today. Only the UVB-spectrum of sunlight, falling directly on the skin, will enable its production in its active form in a sufficient amount. The intestines resorb it only to a small degree. At low altitudes (below 1,200 metres above sea level), sunlight only contains the full UVB spectrum during the summer months, since it is absorbed in the vapour layers when the sunlight is at a low angle of incidence to the surface of the earth. Sun blockers, including those with a very low protection factor, cut out precisely that spectrum of the sunlight. Therefore more frequent exposure to the sun with the head covered but without sun blocker, for a duration of 20 minutes for each side of the body in the summer months, is particularly important for storing the greatest possible amount of vitamin D in the liver as a stock for the winter months.

Vitamin-D substitution reduces the depots of β-amyloid in the inter-cellular tissue of the brain and thus protects against Alzheimer's disease[89]. An increasing number of epidemiological studies indicates that vitamin-D deficiency is associated with a large number of different neuropsychiatric and neurodegenerative diseases[90], including multiple sclerosis[91, 92].

We have seen that there are many diverse causes for neurodegenerative diseases. However, only a few rare cases have genetic causes. In most – and particularly in the most common neurodegenerative diseases, such as multiple sclerosis, Parkinson's disease, Alzheimer's disease and amyotrophic lateral sclerosis – experts cannot reach agreement, since these diseases always have multiple causes and researchers usually deal with them one at a time. More and more scientific evidence for the relevance for neurodegenerative diseases of widespread poor nutrition (i.e. industrially synthesised food high in sugar, white flour, animal fats and proteins, but low in polyunsaturated fatty acids and vegetarian fresh food, in combination with alcohol, coffee and other stimulants) has been collected in recent years. Its relevance is surely still considerably underestimated, however. The causative relevance of many neurotoxins has been thoroughly researched, while the causative relevance of radiation stress will probably become evident in the next few years. The relevance of an orderly lifestyle adjusted to the biological requirements of human life, as well as orderly sleep, is also still greatly underestimated, even though the effect of stress, harassment and bullying and other mental traumas as causative factors for neurodegenerative diseases has already been researched in a neuropsychiatric context.

Assuming a multifactorial cause of such severe diseases, the only possible way to prevent and – where still possible – heal them is to include all causative factors that can be influenced within the treatment plan. This book is based on this insight and on many decades of experience of a very successful treatment of multiple sclerosis and the efficient prevention of other neurodegenerative diseases.

The various types of neurodegenerative diseases

All known neurodegenerative diseases are listed here systematically to provide an overview. Most of these conditions are rare congenital diseases. This book will focus only on multiple sclerosis, Parkinson's disease and amyotrophic lateral sclerosis, in which genetics play no or only a minor role. However, the therapeutic measures described in this book can influence the progress and condition of patients positively even in genetically caused neurodegenerative diseases. In addition, the neurodegenerative diseases with a focus on dementia, their prevention and early treatment, are described in Bircher-Benner manual no. 24: Manual for Prevention of Dementia and Alzheimer's Disease.

Systematic overview of neurodegenerative diseases

Diseases resulting from destructive degenerative proteins: (TAU proteins)
– Alzheimer's disease (AD)
– Progressive supranuclear palsy (PSP)
– Corticobasal degeneration (CBD)
– Argyrophilic grain disease (AGD)
– Frontotemporal dementia, Parkinsonism of the chromosome 17 (FTDP17)
– Pick's disease

Synucleinopathies:
– Parkinson's disease (PD)
– Lewy body dementia (LBD)
– Multiple system atrophy (MSA)

TDP-34 Proteinopathies:
– Frontotemporal lobe degeneration with TDP 34

FUS pathies:
– Frontotemporal lobe degeneration with FUS (FTDL-FUS)
– Neuronal intermediate filament inclusion disease (NIFID)
– Basophilic inclusion body disease (BIBD)

Trinucleotide diseases:
Huntington's disease (HD)
– Spinal and bulbar muscular atrophy, Kennedy type (SBMA)
– Friedreich's ataxia (FA)
– Spinocerebellar ataxia (SCA)
– Dentatorubro-pallidoluysian atrophy (DRPLA)

Prion diseases:
– Creutzfeldt-Jakob disease
– Gerstmann-Sträussler-Scheinker syndrome
– Fatal familial insomnia
– Kuru

Diseases of the motor neurons:
– Amyotrophic lateral sclerosis (ALS)
– Primary lateral sclerosis
– Spinal muscular atrophy (SMA)

Neuroaxonal dystrophies:
– Infantile neuroaxonal dystrophy Seitelberger
– Neurodegeneration with brain iron accumulation (NBIA)

Unclassifiable neurodegenerative diseases:
– Frontotemporal lobe degeneration with ubiquitin proteasome system (FTLD-UPS)

- Familiar encephalopathy with neuroserpin inclusions
- CANVAS (Cerebellar ataxia neuropathy, vestibular areflexia syndrome)

Multiple sclerosis

Parkinson's disease

Amyotrophic lateral sclerosis

Guillain-Barré syndrome

Peripheral neuropathies

Multiple sclerosis

Multiple sclerosis (MS), also called encephalomyelitis disseminata (ED), is a chronically inflammatory disease in which, as we have seen, it is the marrow sheaths or myelin sheaths, the insulating and protective layers around the fast-conducting nerve fibres in the central nervous system, which are attacked. The cause has been the subject of a considerable amount of research and discussion. In young adults, it is one of the most common neurological diseases, along with epilepsy. It causes great suffering among the patients and their families, and it is of considerable socio-medical relevance.

In central Europe, multiple sclerosis is the most common chronically inflammatory disease of the central nervous system. It is about twice as common in women as it is in men. According to current estimates, the frequency (prevalence) of the disease in Germany is 149 patients per 100,000 residents. This means that today about every 750th German is suffering from this disease[93].

The geographic distribution of multiple sclerosis in the world is highly relevant for understanding its causes. In Africa and Central America only 15–18 per 100,000 persons are suffering from disability due to MS. In India, Thailand and Mexico, the numbers are 18–21 patients per 100,000 residents; in Argentina and Australia, 27–30 patients per 100,000 residents; in Europe and Russia, 36–39; in France, Sweden, Norway, Denmark and parts of central Europe, 39–42; and in North America and Alaska, 42–45 per 100,000 residents. It is particularly noticeable that there is a high prevalence in Greenland, with more than 45 persons with disabilities from MS per 100,000 residents (i.e. approx. every two thousandth resident of the country).

People who moved from high-MS zones to low-MS zones as children or in their teens (e.g. from Europe to South Africa or from North America and Europe to Israel) will acquire the disease risk of the target country, while older persons keep the disease risk of their country of origin. This finding is regarded as an important indicator that significant environmental factors in childhood and youth can lead to multiple sclerosis in the adult.

In multiple sclerosis, multiple inflammatory demyelination foci appear scattered throughout the white substance of the brain and spinal cord in which the body's own defence cells and activated oligodendrocytes (turned into macrophages) participate in the maintenance of a massive destructive inflammation in the myelin sheath. Among scientists, whether this is a cause or a consequence of degenerative changes to the lipids (fats) in the myelin sheaths is open to discussion.

Since demyelination foci may appear anywhere in the central nervous system, multiple sclerosis can produce nearly any neurological symptoms. Visual impairment with reduced visual acuity (retrobulbar neuritis) and impairment of the eye movement (internuclear ophthalmoplegia) are typical of multiple sclerosis, but cannot serve as evidence, since they can also have other causes. Multiple sclerosis often causes severe disability relatively late after the disease has appeared. Most of the patients are still able to walk many years after the first neurological symptoms appear. The severity of the disability is often indicated based on a scale (EDDS).

The disease was first described in the Middle Ages, but it was not until 1868 that the French physician Jean Marie Charcot described the symptoms of the disease in detail and coined the term 'Sclérose en plâques'. The pathologist can find focal inflammatory demyelation foci in the white substance in more than one place in the central nervous system. Histologically there is an increased occurrence of glial cells and foci permeated with inflammatory cells in the white substance. The myelin of the marrow sheaths is broken down in the inflammatory foci until only the naked axon (nerve protrusion) is exposed, which will then also be attacked until it is destroyed.

In the first phases of the disease, the ability of the glial cells to repair the marrow sheaths (remyelination), which will cause the neurological symptoms to recede again, is still clearly evident. Remyelinisation by the glial cells is defective, but sufficient for correct nerve conduction. If it succeeds, remyelination can prevent the axon from being destroyed and complete and permanent paralysis from setting in. In the state of demyelinisation, the nerve fibres (axons) only continue to conduct nerve impulses very slowly; as long as they are not destroyed, however, the paralysis can recede when the glial cells regain a thin (but still insulating) myelin layer. Symptoms such as paralysis or visual problems can then still become less severe or disappear entirely. In the later progression, however, permanent paralysis will increase to the same extent as to that at which the axons are destroyed. However, axon damage and permanent paralysis from the very beginning is possible even with the presence of intact myelin sheaths.

Multiple sclerosis usually starts with episodic occurrences of the disease that cause failure symptoms. There is also a rarer variety that is chronically progressive from the beginning. In any case, a chronically progressive disability develops over time. Clinical observation has shown that chronically progressive disability is not directly connected to acute episodes, but rather that chronically progressive disability is due to direct damage to the grey substance during the disability's progress, i.e. the nerve cells (neurons) directly[94].

Pathological anatomic examinations show that there are already diffuse pathological changes even in apparently intact white brain substance when viewed under the microscope[95]. If the demyelinisation has already spread further, the grey substance, where the nerve cells are located, will already present a reduction in the number of brain cells (neurons) by one-fifth, as compared to a healthy cerebral cortex. The loss of neurons may occur before clinical MS symptoms appear. This may continue even after there has been clinical improvement in the disease.

Contrary to former assumptions, new MRI methods such as magnetisation transfer imaging (MTR) show that the destruction of neurons occurs not only in individual lesions, but also diffusely throughout the central nervous system[96].

Causes of multiple sclerosis

The cause is multifactorial, which means that many causes must coincide for the disease to break out. These are the following:

Genetics

There is agreement that MS is not a hereditary disease, even though many genetic mutations have been found in persons suffering from MS. Many of these mutations are directly connected to the immune system, e.g. variants of the tumour necrosis factor 1 gene or genes that are involved in the interleukin signal path. Some of these mutations have also been found in type I diabetes mellitus or Crohn's disease[97, 98, 99, 100, 101], however, but in such a way that their significance is not entirely clear. Examinations of the entire human genome for MS-related genes led to the conclusion that genetics only make up a very small part of the risk of suffering from MS. Most of the gene loci found concerned immune response proteins[102].

Even though reports on various varieties (phenotypes) of multiple sclerosis have been found in India and compared to those in Western countries, more recent studies have shown that the disease makes essentially the same progress in both locations[103]. In identical twins of a parent with MS, the risk that one of the children also develops MS is about 35 %, in siblings about 4 %, in relatives of the 1st degree about 3 %, in relatives of the 2nd degree 1 % and in relatives of the 3rd degree 0.9 %.

The infection hypothesis

For a long time, there was a futile search for a pathogen that caused MS immunologically. Adopted and step children of a person suffering from MS have no increased risk of developing MS, however. Several studies were conducted to clearly exclude a contagious factor of MS[104]. Certain viruses weaken the immune system in general, however, and this may facilitate the development of multiple sclerosis. Some of these are the Epstein-Barr virus and herpes viruses. Children with MS have an Epstein-Barr level in their blood serum more often than other children[105, 106]. This has recently been confirmed for adults as well. Degenerative inflammation of the optical nerve (neuromyelitis optica) occurs more often in multiple sclerosis patients during reactivation of an infection with the Epstein-Barr virus than without this infection[107]. Increased synthesis of antibodies to the Epstein-Barr virus was also found in the brain fluid of patients in early stages of MS, when episodes can still recede entirely[108].

Bacterial infections with chlamydia, spirochetes, rickettsia and streptococcus mutans have been considered triggers of MS. Mycobacterium avium of the sub-species of paratuberculosis (avian tuberculosis) is not only associated with many different diseases in which the autoimmune response plays a role, such as Morbus Crohn, diabetes type 1, sarcoidosis (Morbus Boeck) and autoimmune hashimoto's thyroiditis, but also with multiple sclerosis[109]. On the other hand, there are fewer

MS cases in families with several children under six years of age. This can be explained by the fact that children pass on diseases from one to the other, which tends to strengthen their immune systems[110].

Infections activate interleukins (messenger substances between white blood corpuscles), which can pass the blood-brain barrier on into the nervous system and act on the microglia cells there, so that these will produce additional inflammation mediators (interleukins). It is feasible that infections can trigger MS if the brain is already damaged by neurodegenerative processes caused by poor nutrition, neurotoxins and oxidative stress.

Vitamin D and MS

High levels of vitamin D in the blood reduce the risk of developing multiple sclerosis[111]. Several major studies led scientists to suspect that measures that guarantee an above average vitamin D level would prevent numerous cases of multiple sclerosis[112, 113, 114]. More and more epidemiological studies show that a vitamin D deficit is associated with a wide range of neuropsychiatric diseases[115]. Thus it has also been found in Alzheimer's dementia that a high vitamin D level reduces the deposits of β-amyloids in the connective tissue of the brain[116]. Several scientific works led to the conclusion that vitamin D is a potent natural regulator of the immune system against inflammation. New studies have shown that there are various types of genetically defined vitamin D receptors, though we do not know yet what this means with regard to vitamin D deficiency[117].

Mercury exposure and multiple sclerosis

Many studies from around the world warn of the dangers of mercury.
As described above, amalgam fillings are 50 % composed of liquid mercury. The US Food and Drug Administration (FDA) now warns against use of amalgam[118].
In 1978, a comparative study already documented the fact that persons with amalgam fillings have a higher mortality rate in comparison to a group of people without such fillings[119]. US dentists suffer from multiple sclerosis more often than the norm, since they have to use amalgams with their patients and also often suffer from a very disturbing tremor that is caused by their mercury poisoning (tremor mercurialis)[120]. Persons with amalgam fillings have higher values for mercury vapours in their oral cavities than patients without amalgam fillings. After chewing gum, these values increase 15.6 times[121].

MS patients have more caries and more amalgam fillings than patients without MS, which means that the geographic distribution of caries also matches that of MS[122]. MS patients with amalgam fillings have lower blood cell values than MS patients who have had their amalgam fillings removed, i.e. a lower haemoglobin value and a lower count of T-lymphocytes and CD-8 suppressor cells[123]. Two hundred and seventeen MS patients had increased values of lead from amalgams in MS associated genes, as compared to 496 patients without MS[124].

MS patients have higher average mercury levels in their blood than the group under comparison without MS[125].

It has been scientifically demonstrated that the continuous slow retrograde penetration of methylmercury from amalgam fillings into the roots to the teeth and the body can cause multiple sclerosis[126]. In a comparative study, the hair analyses of MS patients revealed a much higher mercury content than the group in the comparison without MS. MS patients with amalgam fillings also had many and significantly more bouts of the disease than those without amalgam[127].

The liquid metal mercury introduced with the amalgam evaporates at room temperature and when chewing and is organically bound into the body's metabolism, by which it is mostly converted into highly toxic methylmercury. This connects with various other metals and produces allergic reactions. Only chelation removes methyl mercury from the body[128]. In the brain fluid (liquor cerebrospinalis) of MS patients with amalgam fillings, the mercury concentrations were eight times higher than in MS patients without amalgam.

The lymphocytes reactivity test (MELISA) demonstrated that patients with multiple sclerosis or other autoimmune-related diseases have a much increased allergic reaction of their lymphocytes towards different metals and that this metal allergy to mercury and other metals is reduced after the amalgam fillings are removed[129]. The composition of the proteins in the brain fluid (protein electrophoresis of the liquor cerebrospinalis) changed positively and in a dramatic way in MS patients after their amalgam fillings were removed, as compared to the values before amalgam removal[130].

It is very important to note that highly toxic, organically bound methyl mercury is absorbed mainly through food, and mainly by eating mercury-containing fish. Ten percent of the mercury remaining in the body after eating fish is converted into inorganic mercury and partially excreted again via the kidneys, which are then subject to a high level of toxic stress. Part of the mercury from the fish consumed remains in the body, however. Mercury poisoning from eating fish can be best documented through hair analysis. Most fish products, but particularly preserved fish such as tuna, salmon and anchovies, are heavily contaminated with mercury. Additionally, fish are now contaminated with radioactive isotopes from nuclear disasters, nuclear tests and the irresponsible disposal of radioactive waste in the oceans which is then spread throughout all the oceans of the world by the strong ocean currents. The radioactive contamination of food is not really supervised at all for the present, and tinned tuna from the area of Fukushima is sold freely on the global market just as if nothing had happened. For the same reason, we can no longer recommend using sea salt .

Scientific basics for nutritional therapy in multiple sclerosis

For more than 100 years, patients with multiple sclerosis have been treated successfully in the Bircher-Benner centre by detoxing, with an orderly lifestyle, and with an energetically high-quality, essentially vegan diet comprising a large quantity of fresh, raw food and a high content of high-quality lipids and vital substances. If the dietary provisions are complied with, there are usually no more bouts of the disease and the chronic deterioration ends. The prerequisite for this is that all toxic causes, particularly exposure to mercury, are removed at the very beginning of the therapy. Patients with multiple sclerosis have also been treated with a similar diet, orderly lifestyle and naturopathic medicine in other centres since the middle of the last century. One of these is the centre of Dr. Joseph Evers[131].

After decades of a search focused on potential infectious causes for multiple sclerosis, scientific work on the relevance of nutrition as the cause of multiple sclerosis that confirms our dietetic treatment as it is presented in this book has been growing more frequent in recent years.

Table salt and multiple sclerosis
A high consumption of salt increases disease activity and thus accelerates the progress of the disease and worsens the prognosis for curing multiple sclerosis[132, 133]. Table salt inhibits the suppressive function of FOX-P3+ regulating T-lymphocytes and thus promotes inflammatory processes[134].

Animal-based food, plant-based lipids (fats) and multiple sclerosis
Food rich in saturated animal fats increases the risk of developing MS and reduces the progress after the disease breaks out[135, 136, 137, 138, 139, 140]. The earlier in life a diet low in animal fats is started, the lower the risk of developing MS[141]. Supplementation of nutrition with polyunsaturated fatty acids (omega-3 fatty acids) reduces the risk of developing MS considerably[142, 143]. A placebo-controlled comparative study with hospitalised MS patients showed that reduction of animal fats together with the concurrent administration of polyunsaturated omega-3 oils reduced the inflammation parameters of C-reactive protein (CRP), interleukin IL-6 and iso-prostan 8-iso-PGF2a as well as the activity of catalase, as a sign of reduction in inflammations and oxidative stress[144].

Obesity and multiple sclerosis
Obesity increases the risk of multiple sclerosis and is associated with an increased homocysteine level in the blood as a sign of increased risk of neurodegenerative diseases, dementia and multiple sclerosis[145, 146].

Further studies on nutrition and the risk of developing multiple sclerosis
In Gorski Kotar (Croatia), many more people develop multiple sclerosis than in other parts of the same country. This is explained by the high consumption there of whole milk, potatoes with salmon, and fresh or smoked meat[147]. In Ferrara, it was found in a retrospective case-controlled study that persons who were fed large quantities of white bread, pastry, butter,

salmon, vegetable soup, horse meat, coffee and tea in childhood and youth were at greater risk of multiple sclerosis later in life[148]. MS patients with the secondary progressive form of MS had a deficit of folic acid, magnesium, iron and calcium in their nutrition, as compared to the overall population in Holland[149].

Overweight patients with multiple sclerosis, who have large quantities of animal fat in their food, smoke, are socially isolated and treated with interferon, suffer from depression more often than a patient group which regularly takes vitamin D and flaxseed oil, limits alcohol consumption and uses therapeutic counselling (mediation)[150].

A large number of scientific studies have shown that nutrition in the style of western industrialised countries with large quantities of table salt, animal fat, red meat, sugary drinks, roasted and fried food, a deficit of fibre and insufficient physical activity increases the risk of developing MS and negatively impacts the illness' course and prognosis. Such nutrition damages the intestinal environment and its mucosa, and leads to a putrefaction-producing, pathologically changed intestinal flora, to impairment and damage to the enteral immune system (immune system of the intestine), and to the increased production of inflammatory mediators and a tendency to develop chronic inflammation, autoimmune reactions and multiple sclerosis. Nutrition based on fruit and vegetables, on the other hand, is highly effective in preventing multiple sclerosis and improves the patient's progress[151,152,153,154,155,156].

Intestinal milieu, intestinal flora and multiple sclerosis
The great importance of the impaired intestinal flora (intestinal miscolonisation, dysbiosis) and the enteral immune system (immune system of the intestinal mucosa), in addition to subsequent food incompatibilities and food allergies was pointed out early in the 20th century and again in the 1950s. Only recently have research efforts returned to this area[157,158,159]. Thus impaired intestinal flora is considered a highly relevant cause of multiple sclerosis today, since metabolites of certain healthy intestinal bacteria are important for the nervous system and the lack of these bacteria can promote neurological diseases, such as MS[160].

Oxidative stress, antioxidants, omega-3 fatty acids and multiple sclerosis
Regular ingestion of coenzyme Q10, an important antioxidant for the mitochondria, improved various inflammation markers in MS-patients[161,162]. Even a daily supplement of 1.2 mg α-liponic acid as an antioxidant improved the cytokine profile in MS-patients, as a sign of improvement of the inflammatory situation in the immune system, including the parameters INFγ, ECAM-1, TGF-β, IL-4[163]. With high doses, the omega-3 oils improved the disability status. The pi in food must be at least 1:5, but should be 1:1. The positive effect of an increased intake of omega-3 fatty acids led to the conclusion that the impaired omega-6 fatty acid metabolism in MS patients led to the loss of the long chain of omega-6-fatty acids in the myelin sheaths and thus reduced the inflammation-inhibiting cytokine TGF-β, which is promoted by omega-3 fatty acids, in particular in the phase between episodes[164]. In a double blind study with 75 hospitalised MS patients in London and Belfast, those who received plant-based linoleic acid and linolenic acid (flaxseed oil) as a food supplement for two years suffered fewer relapses. The episodes were also less severe than in the comparison group[165]. The same was confirmed in several double blind studies[166,167].

MS patients have increased levels of super oxide radicals (R.O.S.) in the blood[168,169].

This is confirmation that these patients suffer from oxidative stress. In a comparative study of 29 patients with recurring MS episodes (RRMS) and a randomised comparison group without MS, the concentrations of various important parameters for oxidative stress and some antioxidants were measured. The values for enzymes δ-aminolevulinic acid dehydratase and catalase (CAT) were increased; by contrast, the SOD (superoxyd dismutase) was reduced. The researchers found much higher lipid peroxidation and increased carbonyl protein values in the serum of the MS patients. The white blood corpuscles (leucocytes) of MS patients also showed damaged DNA (hereditary material). Additionally, the values for vitamin C, vitamin E, NPSAH and vitamin D in the group of patients with recurring MS episodes were lower than in the healthy control group. These findings show that the oxidative stress in MS patients is high and very relevant, that it attacks the hereditary material and that MS-patients suffer from a lack of important antioxidative vitamins[170]. In another comparative study, patients with recurring multiple sclerosis episodes showed excessively low values of selenium, glutathione peroxidase and the entire range of antioxidants[171].

The myelin of the nerve sheaths contains 20 % cholesterol. This is integrated into the myelin sheaths at low-density lipoproteins (LDL cholesterol). LDL cholesterol is a very important stabiliser of the cell membranes. LDL cholesterol is absolutely vital. It is the form in which the cholesterol synthesised in the liver is absorbed into all tissues of the body. Cholesterol is essential for stabilising all the cell membranes in the body, including the myelin sheaths of the nerve fibres (axons). Arteriosclerosis is not caused by LDL cholesterol, but partially (and vitally) by LDL cholesterol, which has turned rancid (i.e. oxidised) on the way from the liver to the arterial walls in the organism because of a lack of polyunsaturated fatty acids in its lipoprotein molecule. It has been proven that the cholesterol in the myelin sheaths has also turned rancid in multiple sclerosis, so that oxidised LDL cholesterol will be found in myelin sheaths as well as in the arterial walls. In both diseases, this oxidation occurs because of oxidative stress, from the effect of free radicals (R.O.S.), due to a deficit of antioxidative substance in the food[172].

Lack of sleep, melatonin and multiple sclerosis
It has been found that the sleeping hormone melatonin of the epiphysis plays an important role in the development of multiple sclerosis. It could be shown in mice that melatonin prevents cell death (apoptosis) in the central nervous system and improves the movement behaviour of mice. Melatonin improved neurological deficits and paralysis and protects the brain cells (neurons) from destruction. However, melatonin did not lead to a new production of myelin in the marrow sheaths of the nerve fibres[173, 174].

The complexity of causes of multiple sclerosis
It has been shown that the immunological occurrences in the process of self-destruction of the myelin sheaths in multiple sclerosis is much more complex than was long assumed, and that not only the CD-4 helper cells and an impaired ratio of the CD-4-TH1 to the CD-4-TH-2-helper cells are at fault for the uncontrolled inflammation, but that CD-8-suppressor cells, antibody-producing B-cells and microglia cells that convert to macrophages also affect the destructive autoimmune occurrences. Some scientists have come to the conclusion that environmental risk factors such as vitamin D deficit, Epstein-Barr virus infection, smoking, the typical Western diet and an impaired intestinal flora promote the development of multiple

sclerosis in that they interact with genetic mutations to result in a massive regulation impairment of the immune system of the MS patients, which in the end causes self-destruction of the myelin sheaths[175].

On the basis of a year-long randomised controlled comparison study with and without diet[176], the US neurologists' society now recommends a low-fat diet based on fruit and vegetables for all patients suffering from multiple sclerosis. In the meantime, there has been a number of studies that document the positive effects of a vegan diet with addition of omega-3 fatty acids and vitamin D for multiple sclerosis patients[177]. The currently available scientific studies confirm the diverse causes of multiple sclerosis.

According to our experience, the diversity of these causes of multiple sclerosis is in the poisoning with mercury and other neurotoxins, oxidative stress that the patients suffer from, the more or less poor nutrition of these people with a deficit of vital substances, folic acid, vitamins C, D and E, lack of energetically high-quality, fresh, plant-based food with a high content of all anti-oxidative secondary plant substances, a disorderly life, insufficient sleep before midnight and lack of movement.

Remedying these causes is the prerequisite for prevention and, while still possible, for the healing of multiple sclerosis.

It is always impressive to see how this causative treatment and the diet work. The autoallergic inflammation subsides quickly. The impaired microbiological milieu in the intestine, created by poor nutrition and often exacerbated by frequent antibiotic treatments, will be improved within months. We supplement omega-3 fatty acids in the form of biologically produced cold-pressed flaxseed oil, which also contains a large quantity of vitamin E. Vitamins A, C, D, B_6 and B_{12} as well as the selenium level, must be monitored and often require substitutes. All of these values should be brought to the upper standard level. Raw food is rich in folic acid. Nevertheless, the homocysteine level must be monitored and often folic acid must be supplemented at the beginning. Low-level infections such as the Epstein-Barr virus or herpes viruses may flare up in moments of weakness and case deterioration. However, if our diet is strictly followed, such reactivations are very rare.

Food incompatibilities cause inflammation from the formation of inflammation mediators (interleukins).

These promote the autoimmune inflammation in the central nervous system. IgG4-antibody testing can be used to record these. Our experience shows that it is very important to adjust the diet plan specifically to these incompatibilities in order to avoid allergic inflammatory reactions.

Progresses of multiple sclerosis

Without any effective treatment, this disease progresses episodically, followed by slow, persistent deterioration. An episode is defined as the occurrence of new clinical symptoms or the flaring up of old ones that last for more than 24 hours. Every episode is caused by new inflammatory demyelating damage to the myelin sheaths. At least 30 days without new symptoms must pass between two episodes for them to be counted separately. An episode can last from a few days up to a few weeks.

Initially, the symptoms after an episode usually disappear again entirely. This is called *complete remission*. Later, new deteriorations are often partially retained *(incomplete remission)*. This shows that the myelin sheaths were destroyed to the point where the nerve fibre inside them, the axon, has been destroyed and recovery is no longer possible. Neurologists speak of a *pseudo episode* when temporary deterioration occurs in the context of an infection (cold) or fever.

Multiple sclerosis has the following forms of progression:
– relapsing-remitting MS (RRMS);
– secondary progressive MS (SPMS);
– primary progressive MS (PPMS).

The severity and intensity of the individual courses can differ greatly from patient to patient. There are very mild but also very severe developments.
Trigger factors (factors triggering the disease) are conditions that increase the probability of a new episode, such as the flu or any other viral infection (e.g. of the gastrointestinal tract). The risk of an episode in pregnancy is much reduced, but much increased in the first three months after giving birth[178].

The primary progressive course of the disease is found in about 15 % of MS patients.

The symptoms of multiple sclerosis

The first episode usually occurs between 15 and 40 years of age. Very often, the first symptoms will disappear again entirely, which shows that the axons of the nerves have not been attacked yet and that remyelination was sufficient to restore nerve conductivity. Later, residual symptoms will remain, since parts of the axons have been destroyed. Initially, visual and sensitivity problems are frequent symptoms. The disease often starts with a single symptom (CIS).

The location of the first lesion can differ significantly. In 15 % of the patients, the disease starts with usually unilateral, strong reduction of visual acuity or a veil over the field of vision, so that patients can scarcely count their own fingers any more. This shows that the optical nerve is affected (retrobulbar neuritis). Light effects and pain in the eyes are frequent. When the optical nerve near the eye is affected, it will shrink (opticus atrophy). The visual acuity usually improves again after 1–2 weeks. It can also return to normal. One third of the patients develop other symptoms in the following years. This includes seeing double or vertigo and insecurity when walking (ataxia), or swinging eye movements when looking to the side (nystagmus). Electrifying (neuralgic) pain in the face (trigeminus neuralgia) is not infrequently bilateral in MS patients and highly distressing. Epileptic seizures are rare. The flow of speech can be impaired later (chanting speech). Eighty percent of patients develop spastic paralysis. Sometimes hemiplegia may appear within hours of impairment of awareness, and without any pain (type of hemiplegic MS). This can disappear again entirely within a few days or weeks. Disturbance of bladder emptying is frequent, especially in the form of a sudden pressing need to urinate; incontinence and sexual function impairment may occur later. When sensitive nerves are affected, there will be general unpleasant sensations (paresthesias), a feeling of numbness and pain, often in the hands, the lower legs and the feet.

The gait is often insecure and at the same time cramped. The Lhermitte sign is typical for MS. When bending the neck energetically forward, there will be a sensation of an electrical discharge down the spine that may reach into the arms and legs. Often patients are initially characterized by an inappropriate euphoria and a lack of self-awareness regarding the tragic aspects of their disease. Patients are easily exhausted, even if no preceding effort has been made.

Diagnosis of multiple sclerosis

Today diagnosis is based on imaging procedures (MR). At least two inflammatory foci in different locations must be documented. Gadolinium-containing contrast agents show the permeability of the blood-brain barrier. The McDonald criteria require that fresh and old foci be visible at the same time. After two episodes in neurologically different systems, the diagnosis can also be made without MR.

There are not always signs of inflammation in the blood in lab examinations. It is still unclear whether the determination of the basic myeloproteine (MBP) and myelin-oligodendrocytes-glycoprotein (MOG) contribute to diagnosis. A spinal tap is more indicative. Every second patient has an increased count of lymph cells. In 95 % of the patients, one can find oligoclonal bands in the isoelectrical focus as an important indication of an inflammatory process in the central nervous system. Eighty-nine percent of patients show evidence of antibody synthesis in the brain for measles, rubella and varicella zoster viruses (MRZ). The lab tests do not permit a clear diagnosis, however. The electroencephalogram (EEG) shows indications of an impaired conduction of stimuli where myelin is damaged, and signs of damage to the nerve fibres (axons) where the amplitude of the electrical potentials is reduced.

Diagnosis of multiple sclerosis is not easy, since various other diseases can imitate its symptoms. These include syphilis, AIDS, neuroborreliose, and autoimmune diseases such as collagenoses and vasculitides (autoimmune vasculitis). Tropical spastic paraparesis or acute disseminated encephalomyelitis (ADEM) and certain metabolic diseases (leucodystrophies) can lead to similar symptoms and findings in magnetic tomography (MR). Certain psychiatric diseases or severe vitamin-B_{12} deficit (funicular myelosis) must also be considered[179].

Medical treatment of multiple sclerosis

Treatment with medication cannot heal the disease, but in the best case can delay its progress by attempting to suppress the immune system in order to delay self-destruction of the nervous system.

Pharmacological treatment of acute episodes

In German-speaking regions, the treatment recommendations are specified in the directives of the 'Multiple Sklerose-Therapie Konsensus-Gruppe' (MSTKG). If only sensation is impaired, treatment with medication is usually dispensed with. This is different when paralysis or visual impairment occurs. The corticosteroids (cortisol, prednisone, prednisolone) inhibit inflammatory processes and can help seal the blood-brain barrier. They inhibit the growth and migration of white blood corpuscles into the brain and it is hoped that they can protect the nerve fibres (axons). To this day, however, there is no scientific proof that these medicines positively influence the long-term course of multiple sclerosis.

As pulse treatment, 1,000 mg of methylprednisolone are usually administrated in the form of infusions over five days. If the symptoms are not much improved after two weeks, there is a second pulse treatment with up to twice the prednisolone dose. Important side effects are sleeping problems and an instable mood.
If the pulse treatment does not reduce the symptoms satisfactorily, plasmaphoresis is considered, especially if there is severe paralysis. In 40 % of all cases, plasmaphoresis can reduce the symptoms[180]. Side effects are infections and disorders of the cardiovascular system, which may also become severe.

Treatment between episodes

The target is to influence the immune system so that the autoimmune inflammation is suppressed. The beta interferons teriflunomide or leflunomide or nazalinumab are regarded as *immunomodulation*. The effects of these medicines are diverse and not fully understood. Nazalinumab is intended to inhibit the migration of white blood corpuscles through the blood-brain barrier. The monoclonal antibody alemtuzumab is to inhibit the congenital immune system (complement system) temporarily.

Azathioprine, cyclophosphamide, fingolimod and mitoxatron are *immunosuppressives*. They reduce the increase in the number of white blood corpuscles and thus partially suppress inflammatory processes in the brain. It is hoped that these medicines may delay the progression of the disease and prevent damage to the nerve fibres (axons).

Pharmacotherapy at the relapsing-remitting course (RRMS)

In the early stage of MS, the inflammatory processes in the central nervous system are particularly severe. Therefore the directives recommend the immediate commencement of an immunomodulation 'basic therapy' either with glatirameracetat or a β-interferon-preparation. If there are any counter-indications for these medicines, azathioprine and intravenous immunglobulins are used instead. If the neurological symptoms still grow worse, 'escalation treatment' with mitoxantron, natalizumab, fingolimod and rarely cyclophosphamide is recommended, even through meta analyses have not found any convincing evidence of the effectiveness of such preparations[182]. This treatment is usually continued for as long as it seems to be effective without any severe side effects. Mitoxantron is particularly dangerous because of its toxic effect on the heart. Antibodies against β-interferon and natalizumab may develop (nAB) and render these medicines ineffective.

The chronically progressive MS
In about 15 % of all patients, MS does not develop in episodes, but rather is chronically progressive from the beginning. Even an initial recurring course of the illnesss will slowly transform itself into a chronic progression with permanent neurological failures. In spite of the high toxicity for the heart (cardiotoxicity), mitaxoantron is used in this case, up to the maximum lifetime dose. Then there will be an attempt to influence the course by surge therapy with highly-dosed quarterly infusions of a corticoid, usually methylprednisolone or cyclophosphamide. However, a multiple sclerosis having a chronic progression from the beginning can hardly be influence by medication.

Supporting symptomatic treatment
Patients suffer most from walking disability, spasticity and pain, speech and swallowing impairment and depression. They will also tire very quickly. Physiotherapy, osteopathy, neural therapy, speech therapy and occupational therapy can help. In the case of marked walking disability, the medicine Fampirin is often used in order to block the potassium canals of the damaged nerves to make it easier to walk[183]. If the large motor-track (tractus pyramidalis) has been damaged by the sclerosis foci, the patients suffer from enormous cramps (spasticity). Physiotherapy works by shutting down neuromuscular reflexes, in this instance according to the Bobath concept. Medicines are often prescribed, including baclofen, tizanidin or injections of botulinus toxin. Cannabis primarily has a cramp-relieving effect, so that tetrahydrocannabinol (THC) has also been permitted for the treatment of strong spasticity. Cannabis sativa at high homeopathic potency is one of the most important homeopathic treatments of multiple sclerosis. Another homeopathic remedy that often has great effect is agaricus muscaris (A high potency from the fly agaric toadstool).

The trigeminus neuralgia (tormenting electrifying pain in the face) is tackled with carbamazepine, gabapentin, pregabalin or amitriptyline in conventional medicine[184]. Neural therapy in the hands of a qualified physician can be a great help here. The patients often suffer from bladder function impairments with infections of the urinary tract, a sudden urge to urinate or incontinence, speech disorders or erectile dysfunction.

Stem cell transplants
Some centres try, similarly to leukaemia, to kill the entire immune system cytostatically and then to introduce stem cells to produce a more tolerant new immune system. This treatment promises little success, since it is not aimed at the cause of multiple sclerosis and entails a high risk for the patients[185].

All of these pharmacological therapeutic approaches attempt to suppress the inflammatory activity of the immune system to delay the relapses of multiple sclerosis and its progression to the disastrous destruction of the nerve axon with permanent paralysis. Unfortunately, these medicines have many side effects, some of which are dangerous, which the patients are exposed to and that often result in the discontinuation of treatment.

Order therapy for multiple sclerosis

The treatment approach described in this book is unique. It is about finding all the recognisable causes and removing them while at the same time very efficiently supporting the regenerative forces so that they can prevail over the destructive processes. This permits permanent repair of the attacked myelin sheaths and prevents new inflammation foci from developing.

We have seen the central relevance of toxic heavy metals and other environmental toxins, and how oxidative stress from a lifestyle contrary to our biological needs plays a central role in multiple sclerosis. We have seen the great causative influence of the typically poor nutrition of multiple sclerosis patients, a nutrition containing large quantities of animal fat, meat, roasted substances, white flour, sugar, coffee, alcohol and other stimulants, in addition to drugs and medicines and a highly significant deficit in vital substances, vitamins D and E, folic acid, omega-3 fatty acids and vegetarian foods containing antioxidative, regenerating phytochemicals. We have seen how oxidative stress promotes inflammation and attacks the sensitive lipids of the nerve sheaths and the blood-brain barrier. We have also seen how the oxidative stress of the patients overburdens the capacity of the antioxidative, regenerating systems until an excessive number of free radicals (R.O.S.) are produced. These R.O.S. attack the myelin sheaths by lipid-peroxidation, thereby harming and destroying them. We have seen how chronic inflammation in the intestine, in the body and in tooth-root foci release interleukins and cause inflammatory processes in the central nervous system to promote and maintain the destructive autoimmune process.

MS patients are often unable to recognise the tragic and dangerous aspects of their disease. They are unable to understand and apply our order treatment. Use of a course of carefully considered, high potency homeopathic treatment chosen by an experienced doctor and adapted to the patient's individual situation can clear the path to the treatment of the causes. Frequently recommended medicines are cannabis indica and agaricus muscaris, which must be used at very high potencies, usually a 100,000th Korsakow potency. However, homeopathy alone cannot heal multiple sclerosis. Diet is decisive.

Order therapy and dietetics will have a considerable effect because of their striking ability to bring about change and regeneration, already even in the first few weeks. Experiencing this is invariably fascinating both for the patients and the doctor on every single occasion. Beginning treatment immediately is decisive for the prognosis. Early diagnosis and consistent detoxing of the organism from any clearly neurotoxic substances are also decisive.

Tooth amalgams and other toxic tooth materials must be removed under very careful protective measures, and then eliminated from the connective tissue, the cells and the central nervous system. Tooth root abscesses cause cadaveric poisons. They must be found and remedied, along with any other infectious sources in the body.

Unhealthy intestinal flora with the accompanying putrefaction and toxins represent an immense interference in the metabolism. If the intestinal milieu is disrupted in this way, maturation of the dendritic cells and lymphocytes of our immune system into immunocompetent cells cannot occur in a reliable fashion. The differentiation between foreign and endogenous becomes uncertain, so that the immune system tends to develop autoimmune reactions. Sensitive nerve endings from the intestinal mucosa also activate the hormonal stress axis via the brain stem, so that the adrenal gland produces too much adrenalin which encourages inflammatory processes.

The only possible way out of this situation is a diet of fresh vegetarian food as described in this book, supported by microbial treatment. Such a diet promotes the settlement of healthy intestinal germs, quickly and noticeably changes the general metabolism, and restores food efficiency. This leads to a strong detoxing effect. The degenerative proteins, amyloids, organic acids and oxidised lipids stored in the basic substance (matrix) of the inter-cell substance of the connective tissue in the brain, in the spinal cord and throughout the body will slowly be reduced and discharged, and the blood-brain barrier will be regenerated.

The entire detoxing process will take months or even years. Strong willpower is needed if the patient is to prevail over multiple sclerosis. The high energy potential of fresh vegetarian food – with its high content in biologically regenerative information and antioxidative, immunomodulating secondary plant substances (phytochemicals), polyunsaturated fatty acids, vitamins and folic acid – causes a general regeneration and relieves the antioxidative systems. The levels of vitamins D, E, B_{12} and folic acid in the blood must be brought to the upper-standard level. To accelerate regeneration of the mitochondria and cell energy, we perform high-dosage infusion treatment with antioxidants for the nervous system, especially in the initial phase, and administer to the patient membrane-effective coenzyme Q10 in its most highly effective form as ubiquinone. This comprehensive treatment will cause the mitochondria to recover quickly and render them able to reproduce again. The patient will soon feel an improvement in cell energy in the form of a new vitality and renewed life energy. He will find new courage and experience a justified hopefulness. The fatigue depression will disappear and make way for a new optimism with which to face the future.

A life style characterized by greater order which includes pre-midnight sleep is also very important. We have seen that the sleeping hormone melatonin from the epiphysis has an important influence on the course of multiple sclerosis. Natural high melatonin levels can be achieved only with at least three hours of sleep before midnight. We fall into the deep, restorative non-rem sleep phases in the hours before midnight. After midnight, we almost only experience restless REM sleep phases with intense dream experiences that serve mental healing, but not restoration and recovery of the neurons of our brains. It is only in the non-REM sleep phases before midnight that our nervous system can recover sufficiently. This recovery is extremely important for healing multiple sclerosis. We have also seen that sufficient activity, sport or hiking in the fresh air positively influences the course of the disease and promotes healing. Exposure to sunlight is also very important for regeneration. It not only results in vitamin D synthesis but also has a direct, positive effect on the nervous system via the melanin metabolism. Body regulation should also be stimulated by alternating hot and cold baths and gushes, air baths and dry brushing. The relationship between multiple sclerosis patients and their families is often characterised by conflict, feelings of guilt, the disease itself, the slow loss of independence, feelings of taking offence, and helplessness. It is easy to feel guilty towards others, and the family feels helpless at being unable to do more. Often one has to learn to see which feelings of guilt are justified and which are not. Once this distinction is made, it is easier for everyone concerned. Justified feelings of guilt can only be relieved by trying to better understand the other's need and to ask for reconciliation for mistakes made. If this does not produce satisfactory results, one must accept outside help.

Supporting measures for nursing of the patient, water applications

As previously described, multiple sclerosis patients suffer from partially spastic and partially limp paralysis, for example of the feet, legs, urinary bladder, arms. These body parts suffer from severely impaired circulation. The inactivity of the muscles due to paralysis in the affected limbs leads to a defective supply with oxygen and nutrients in the muscle tissues, the skin, the nerves, the joints and joint capsules, the ligaments and tendons and the bones (inactivity atrophy). The affected limbs turn cold and blue and are in danger of developing frostbite.

Over time, the cold will spread through the entire body. This makes the patients susceptible to infections of all kinds. The cold also reaches the digestive organs, so that the patients often suffer from flatulence, constipation or diarrhoea. Even if the bladder is not yet paralysed, the lack of circulation in the pelvic organs will make patients susceptible to inflammation of the bladder and the sexual organs.

Two kinds of heat, active and passive warming

External warmth enters the body passively. When the body is thoroughly warm, it can in turn produce active heat as the result of a careful, appropriate cold stimulus that will stimulate the body to react in order to warm itself. This will improve circulation in the affected limbs. In the hands of an experienced therapist hot and cold baths and gushes are simple and highly effective ways for activating the circulation in the affected limbs and organs, and for improving their supply of oxygen and nutrients. The body must always be thoroughly warmed before a cold application, and the stimulus must not be too strong; it must be carefully adjusted to the patient's condition. Under these conditions, alternate hot and cold treatments are a great help for MS patients. They stimulate and maintain the body's own regulative processes and thus prevent atrophy coming from inactivity.

Hydrotherapy for MS patients

The rising-temperature alternating foot bath

One plastic tub should be filled with lukewarm water and a second tub with cold water. Patients' feet should be placed in the warm water (to just above the ankles), then hot water carefully added until they can just bear the heat and a pleasant warmth spreads from the feet throughout the body (take care in case of sensitivity impairment). When patients subsequently wish to cool their feet, they should place them in cold water and leave them there until they feel refreshed and the patients then have the desire to take them out. Patients should at this point dry their feet thoroughly and lie under a warm duvet. This alternating foot bath can be repeated several times per day. In case of excessive general weakness, alternate washes of the feet and legs are to be administered from the very beginning. Patients who are particularly weak may find sitting up on the edge of the bed for the foot bath to be too exhausting. In that case, warming can be achieved with a hot-water bottle or, better, a hay flower bag heated in hot steam. For cooling, patients may apply cold

Preissnitz/Kneipp compresses made by placing a towel in cold water and wringing it out until it is just cold and moist rather than cold and dripping. It should be placed around the foot with a second, dry towel placed over it. Once there are compresses on both feet, patients should be covered up completely. If patients are so weak that the body is scarcely able to produce warmth, hot-water bottles should be placed at the knees, stomach or wherever else they wish. The foot compress stays in place until the patients feel a strong, pleasant warmth in the feet that signals that good circulation has developed in that part of the body.

The alternating lower leg bath
This requires two plastic tubs that are high enough to put the lower legs up to the knees in the water. Proceed as for the alternating foot bath. If the patient is strong enough, he can cool this part of the body whilst standing or sitting in the shower and making use of a shower head. Otherwise, the patient can make use of a cold wash and, when he is stronger, of Preissnitz compresses as for the foot bath.

The alternating hip bath
A hip bath to the navel with a rising temperature can be very helpful as well, with a brief cooling of the middle of the body by washing or with the shower head or, if the necessary equipment is at hand, in the form of alternating hip baths and using two hip bath tubs. Using the bath tub, the patient can place a stool under the knees and lower legs when warming up, then drain off the warm water and apply the cold water with the shower head. The alternating hip bath leads to a thorough internal warming of the pelvic organs, the hips and belly and is also particularly suitable for a weak bladder.

The alternating arm bath
This can be done by sitting in front of the sink and putting the arms into warm water, subsequently draining off this water for the cold application and then briefly applying a cold gush to both arms.

Warm steaming of the head
Steam from an electric kettle is carefully directed at the face with the help of a large bath towel until a pleasant warmth is felt. Cooling takes place using a cold wash.

On a hot summer day or in an overheated apartment, this application does not begin with additional warming, but begins with immediate cooling. For example, the patient can sit briefly in a cold hip bath on a hot day in high summer. Then he should dry off the cooled body parts and return to bed for rest. Equally, cold Kneipp gushes can be applied with a garden hose on hot summer days, as well as cold foot, leg, knee, back, spinal, arm, face, ear or eye gushes. When it is very hot, drying off is not necessary.

Dry brushing
Dry brushing increases circulation through reflex stimuli. You can use a clothes brush that is not too hard or, better, a special brush with a long handle that can be acquired from a medical supply store. The skin warms up pleasantly under the brush and turns red, but should not be painful. If possible, the patient should brush his entire skin in the morning, starting with the hair or the soles of the feet. If the patient cannot reach every part of the body, it is for the caregiver to do this brushing. Invigoration of the skin can bring great relief to multiple sclerosis patients.

Exposig the skin to the sun
We have seen how important an adequate vitamin D level is for preventing and fighting multiple sclerosis. The UVB light spectrums are present in sunlight everywhere in the summer half of the year, but only in the mountains at altitudes above

1200 m in winter. Even very weak sun blockers will completely protect the body from the effect of the UVB light spectrums. Therefore regular exposure to the sun in summer is very important. Only the head should be covered and exposure should last 20 minutes per body side, without a sun blocker. The head should be covered to protect the nerve cells of the brain. Light-haired, pale people are more sensitive and should not spend more than 10 minutes in the sun. In high summer, the sun bath should take place before 10 a.m. or after 3 p.m., since the stimulus of the sun at noon is too strong. MS patients suffering from closed tuberculosis or currently having an infection must not be exposed to blazing sunlight. If you want to stay in the sun for a longer period, apply a fast reacting crystalline sun blocker cream after the time spent unprotected. Sunbathing individual parts of the body is also effective and sensible. Sunbathing not only activates vitamin D that is stocked in the liver for the winter, but also modulates the immune system and promotes the formation of high-energy phosphates.

Solariums do not emit any UVB light. They only produce a fast tan that rapidly fades without any health value and without the production of any vitamin D. Treating the skin with an artificial sunray lamp (medical quartz lamp) is sensible in the winter half of the year and should be done according to precise medical instructions of the specified duration and using protective goggles. It is a good idea to combine the UVB light with a warming infrared lamp. Carbon steam lamps produce the visible medium wave and infrared spectrum of sunlight. This is extremely valuable for the general health as well and can also be performed under a bed light arc, a kind of tunnel with a reflective inner layer with the carbon steam lamps being activated at the top. The bed light bath brings about a pleasant feeling of relaxation in the patients, passive warming and improved circulation, and should be concluded with a brief cold wash or cold gush of various body parts, and a subsequent dry brushing. The patient should then rest, snugly enveloped in blankets.

The air bath
An air bath is a sensible alternative on cooler days or at warm times with a cloud cover.

The great relevance of fresh air
The MS patient should endeavour to breathe clean, fresh air rich in oxygen, day and night. This is mandatory for the regeneration processes in the central nervous system. The bedroom should not face onto a busy street, so that the window can remain open at night without fear of pollution.

Avoiding electro smog and pulsed high-frequency radiation
It is very important that MS patients protect themselves from electro smog caused by mobile phone aerials and house phones where at all possible. It may be necessary and the only sensible thing to find an apartment that permits this. The entire power supply, including cables and lamps, must be properly earthed. Radio alarm clocks, WLAN, other wireless connections and wireless house phones should be replaced by wired connections.

Daily movement
We have seen the great influence of daily movement for the prevention and healing of multiple sclerosis. MS patients should spend as much time as possible hiking in a natural environment, on level ground as well as uphill and downhill. MS patients also should sing as much as possible. The joy and inner elation of the experience of singing will cause cramps to recede. Hiking is medicine for the entire body – the heart, circulation, veins, blood supply,

breathing, digestive organs, joints and particularly the central nervous system – because it stimulates the circulation and the oxygen supply to the brain. Work when sitting and standing puts a considerable strain on the circulation, reduces the blood flow in the brain and increases the risk of thrombosis and embolisms. When hiking, the muscles of the legs also pump blood back to the heart and thus the heart needs to make less of an effort to pump the blood. The better the circulation, the better the nerve cells and nerve sheaths are supplied with blood that is rich in nutrition and oxygen. The MS patient should always adjust his hiking to his own available strength and not attempt to hike beyond his physical abilities. He will reach his goal best through careful, pleasant and incremental effort.

The overheating treatment

We recommend overheating treatment during a relapse of the disease or during infection, as well as each week in winter. Proceed as follows when nursing at home: drink a sufficient quantity of linden blossom or elder tea at 11 a.m. or 3 p.m. while in bed, place several rubber hot-water bottles against your body and see that you are warmly wrapped up. This warms up the whole body and produces a slight fever. If a bedside light-bath is at hand, the patient can achieve this aim even more easily. He should remain in this warm environment for about half an hour. Then, for a few seconds each, the nurse has to wash off one part of the body at a time with cold water. The washed parts are rubbed dry at once and covered with a duvet. Proceed as follows: head with left arm, right arm with chest, belly with left leg and then the right leg with the back. The precise succession of these manipulations is a matter of individual choice. Then, if the patient can tolerate it, the heat treatment and cold wash can be repeated. The immune system is not stimulated by sweating, but by the strong flow of the blood during the warming of the body. Many women, and more rarely men, produce no or little sweat during this treatment. This is not relevant for the effect, since "overheating" is what matters. Under a doctor's supervision, the "overheating" treatment can also be performed with a rising-temperature bath in a bathtub of linden wood, or a regular bath if the heart and circulation permit.

Medical massage

As mentioned, MS patients suffer from partially spastic and partially limp paralysis, so that the muscles threaten to atrophy and the circulation to become impaired. Kneading and stroking massages of the paralysed limbs and the entire body counter this risk. All the skin, muscles, joints, arteries, veins and nerves that are accessible are treated this way. The patient will be able to treat himself as far as his strength permits and depending on how well he can reach the parts of his body. Otherwise the treatment should be performed by memers of the family or nursing staff. The massage technique must be taught by a trained specialist initially. If the massage can be performed under a heat light arc, it will have a much stronger effect. Always follow up with a cold wash, as described above. The legs may be massaged even if the patient has varicose veins, but not if there is any fresh thrombosis. The technique of connective tissue massage, as recommended by Elisabeth Dicke, is also valuable. Today most medical massage therapists master this technique.

Movement exercises

These counter the reduced performance of the nerves, muscles and blood vessels and keep the joints mobile. In the case of paralysed limbs this means passive movement, which a doctor or therapist will teach the members of the family and the patient. The patient should attempt to do as much as possible on his own: loosening up gymnastics and tensioning/relaxing free gymnastics on the bed or on a mat in the room or on the lawn, in the garden, etc. Instructions for this can be requested from the multiple sclerosis associations.

Emptying the intestine

The enema
Patients who are bedridden and no longer able to hike often suffer from difficulties in evacuating the bowels, even though the healing diet at least partially remedies this problem. The dietary instructions in our Bircher-Benner manual no. 14 for patients with gastrointestinal conditions and microbial treatment (symbiosis control) often provide significant help in such cases. If further treatment is necessary, there is no substitute for a lukewarm chamomile tea enema with a large rubber balloon syringe or an intestinal rinsing vessel with a tube (irrigator) carried out at regular intervals. Never use soapy water.

The retained enema
Cold chamomile tea is injected into the rectum with a small rubber balloon syringe in the early morning, just after the patient has woken up. If this leads to an immediate slight urge to empty the bowels, the urge can be easily suppressed by consciously retaining the enema in the rectum. The large intestine is forced to warm the cold liquid of the retained enema, which strongly stimulates the blood circulation in the rectum. This will slowly improve the muscle tone and the strength of the rectum and thus its ability to discharge its contents. Carried out in this way, frequent enemas are sensible and not harmful.

The importance of sleeping before midnight
The restorative non-REM sleep phases with few dreams occur almost only in the time before midnight. During the REM phases of sleep (rapid eye-movement phases) after midnight, we sleep much less deeply. At that time, sleep is characterised by intense dream experiences, which do not serve physical recuperation, though they do contribute to the reprocessing of emotional experiences and so have a beneficial effect on mental health. All muscles other than the heart, diaphragm and the eye muscles are partially paralysed during this time in order to prevent us from getting up and sleepwalking. The phenomena outlined above can in fact be observed in all people and can be defined as our natural sleeping pattern. Those who call themselves 'night owls' live contrary to their own inherent nature and must in the long run expect to suffer from exhaustion and considerable regulation impairment.

The non-REM phases of sleep are very important for successful regeneration in the central nervous system. People suffering from neurodegenerative diseases must go to bed between 7 and 8 p.m. and get up early as a natural consequence. Sleeping late in the morning does not improve their health, though breaks for a rest in the shape of short naps are sensible in the course of the day.

On sexuality during multiple sclerosis
A patient may be allowed to have sex with his usual trusted partner. If the relationship with the partner is healthy, sexual relations will not weaken the patient. On the contrary, they will improve relaxation and their overall equilibrium.

On the general lifestyle with multiple sclerosis

MS is a serious disease. It involves a great deal of worry and usually makes a reduction of the work load imperative. This in turn often confronts the family with considerable financial problems. If such concerns lead to discouragement, sadness and desperation, the healing of multiple sclerosis will only be all the more difficult. Some patients will refuse to reflect on the dangerous and tragic aspects of their disease; they lose their sense of reality and therefore are unwilling even to begin with diet or treatment. As previously mentioned, carefully and individually chosen homeopathic treatment at very high potencies can also be very helpful in such cases.

Healing multiple sclerosis or preventing its progression when permanent paralysis has already occurred is an immense task for the patient and his family, though one that is well worth the effort.
We are capable of growing into the task before us. Understanding and tackling this comprehensive treatment will awaken powerful healing forces in the patient. There will be a deeper inner maturation of the personality. We will begin to see the serious violations which we and our ancestors have come to commit in respect of the natural laws for the order of life and good health. More and more, we will become able to see our previous subjugation to what is deemed modern and contemporary, the relevance for sickness of a previous nutrition contrary to all reason, the nonsense of chasing after money and consumables to the point of exhaustion in the sphere of one's profession, the senseless struggle to acquire what is generally considered to be a higher standard of living, the mental and cultural loss suffered with regard to the real sense of human existence.

Fighting for one's own recovery helps to develop one's insight into multifacetted nature of life in general. This can transform the patient into a potential source for further reflection and emotional development for his family and a larger circle of individuals and can enrich them by so imparting courage and an inner strength through his example. Thus the patient becomes of value to others in a very different, new fashion, in this technological age characterized by the twilight of all that is human and humane, with its superficial and of necessity distorted manifestations of what are made to appear to be the ideas of the majority. We specifically refer to the book *Vom Werden des neuen Arztes (The Physician of the Future)*, by Dr. med. Maximilian Bircher-Benner here. Reading it will certainly give some encouragement to anyone suffering from multiple sclerosis, and will hopefully do the same for the family of the patient, too.

The relationship with art is to be deepened and the works chosen carefully. Regarding literature, Shakespeare's "Hamlet" and his Sonnets are masterpieces, and the poems of Keats and Wordsworth are also very suitable. Dickens' "David Copperfield" and "A Christmas Carol" are excellent, as are the works of the Americans Longfellow and Emerson. They can be a great help in furthering one's own awareness. Music should be chosen carefully, too. The works by Beethoven, Bach, Haydn, Schubert and Brahms are particularly helpful, while other composers – especially modern ones – and contemporary popular music flood us with the rather irrelevant zeitgeist (the spirit of the age) and further dissonance. The inner conflict produced by such music is detrimental to healing. Choosing artistic masterpieces by Rembrandt, Albrecht Dürer, Albert Anker, Raffael, Michelangelo, Rodin and the great impressionists and looking at them frequently is also a very rewarding occupation.

Goethe wrote in 'Faust II': 'This is the ultimate truth: Only those who have to fight for it every day, deserve to live their lives in true freedom. This means the freedom from our own emotional weaknesses and imperfection, and freeing oneself from the current types of thought and action.

If someone becomes ill and requires nursing, relationships in the family and with relatives will be put to the test. Much has been said, preached and written about love. When someone asks what love actually is, we often do not know the right answer. Mathias Claudius, the famous German poet, once wrote: 'We are not at home where we have our domicile, but where we are understood.' We trust those who understand us. We deserve trust when we understand others. The many suffering people we have met in our consultations have been our greatest teachers. They have taught us that love cannot be anything other than understanding and being understood. When we understand a suffering person, we love him. When others understand us, we are loved. If we manage to understand ourselves, we are able to recognise, honour and love ourselves.

Parkinson's disease

Parkinson's disease is also called idiopathic Parkinson syndrome (IPS), shaking palsy or paralysis agitans. Parkinson's disease results from the slowly progressing death of the nerve cells in the substantia nigra, a nerve ganglion of the midbrain which is responsible for activating the movement processes controlled by the cerebrum. The nerve cells of the substantia nigra produce the activating neurotransmitter dopamine. A lack of dopamine reduces the activating effect of the basal ganglia of the extrapyramidal motoric system on the cerebral cortex.

Recent research on the rare congenital forms of Parkinson's syndrome have shown that this is not one consistent disease, but an entire group of clonal and pathological varieties (PARK 1 to PARK 13). Genetically caused forms are only responsible for 5–10 % of all cases of Parkinson's disease, among them specifically point mutations of the α-synuclein gene (SNCA-gene, PARK 1), in which α-synucleine (SNCA) is evident in the LEWY-bodies in the substantia nigra. A-synuclein has been connected with the formation of fibrillar aggregates that destroy the nerve cells[186, 187]. Several studies have found indications that various versions of the SNCA-gene are associated with sporadic Parkinson's syndrome[188]. Today, more than every hundredth person above sixty is affected by this serious neurodegenerative disease.

Parkinson's disease causes the nerve cells in the pars compacta of the substantia nigra (Latin for 'black substance') in the midbrain to die. These nerve cells produce dopamine and transport it through their nerve fibres (axons) into the brain stem ganglion putamen. The first symptoms will not occur before 55 % of the neurons in the substantia nigra have been destroyed. The messenger substances glutamate and acetylcholine are predominant where there is a deficit of dopamine. The globus pallidus internus should be activated by the dopamine from the substantia nigra and in turn activate the cerebral cortex via the thalamus. Since the activity in the globus pallidus is too weak because of a lack of dopamine, the motoric cerebral cortex is inhibited. This leads to the characteristic symptoms of Parkinson's disease: marked trembling (tremor, 'pill-turning tremor'), general stiffness (rigor) and abrupt slowing of the movements (hypokinesia and cogwheel phenomenon), as well as a general slowing of all mental processes (bradyphrenia). In addition to the dopamine deficit, Parkinson's disease is also characterized by changes to other messenger substances (neurotransmitters) in other brain regions, such as a deficit of serotonin, acetylcholine and noradrenalin[189].

The causes of Parkinson's disease

Toxins have been identified as the causes. Toxic metals such as mercury from tooth fillings with amalgams and consumption of fish such as salmon, tuna and anchovies[190, 191, 192, 193, 194, 195, 196], as well as aluminium, cadmium, copper[197, 198, 199, 200], zinc, manganese, iron and arsenic[201, 202, 203, 204, 205]. Furthermore, some pesticides[206, 207, 208, 209, 210, 211, 212, 213, 214] and metal-based nanoparticles have been identified as causes of Parkinson's disease[215, 216, 217]. Pesticides such as Paraquat, Rotenon, Lindane and Dieldrin activate the microglia, the immune system of the brain, in different ways through activation of NADPH-oxidase (NOX 2)[218]. It also has been documented that such environmental effects during pregnancy and in early childhood will act on the genes to favour the development of neurodegenerative diseases later in life[219, 220, 221, 222]. This disease can occur even at younger ages in case of stress from toxic metals or pesticides[223]. These environmental toxins encourage the formation of β-amyloid and phosphorylisis of TAU-proteins in the brain, which lead to the senile amyloid plaques in Alzheimer's disease and the formation of twisted fibrils that destroy the nerve cells. In Alzheimer's disease, the toxic effects of lead, manganese, solvents and certain pesticides are considered responsible for the destruction of the mitochondria and the disturbed metal metabolism and the aggregation of degenerative proteins, among others the α-synuclein, which destroys the nerve cells in the substantia nigra that should produce DOPAMINE to maintain correct movement control by development of LEWY-bodies[224, 225]. In this degenerative process, oxidative stress is a decisive factor[226, 227, 228, 229, 230]. Coenzyme Q10 helps with the phosphorylation of the high-energy phosphates in the chemical respiratory chain of glucose degradation, and thus improves the cell energy in the nerve cells[231]. In the 1980s, many young people in California injected the opium drug Pethidine, which was contaminated with MTPP (1-Methyl-4-phenyl-1,2,5,6-Tetrahydropyridin). They quickly developed severe toxic Parkinson's syndrome. MPTP is converted into the highly toxic molecule MPP+ (1-methyl-4-Phenylpyridin) in the brain. The molecule MPP is similar enough to dopamine to enter the nerve cells (neurons) of the substantia nigra via the dopamine transport system and to destroy them[232, 233, 234]. The molecule of the common herbicide Paraquat is similar to MPP+ in its structure. Studies from Canada have shown that areas where Paraquat was used have an above-average frequency of Parkinson's disease[235]. Another pesticide that produces Parkinson's disease is the insecticide Rotenone. In animal studies, it could be shown that Rotenone causes discharge of α-synuclein (SNCA), which is a protein produced in the body that, similar to MPP+, has a toxic effect at the dopaminergic nerve cells and causes them to degenerate[236]. Phenol compounds are neurotoxic. They pass unhindered through the blood-brain barrier and may cause severe neurodegenerative damage. They are still permitted in the cosmetics industry and contained in innumerable shower and bath additives, ointments and creams. In France, Parkinson's disease is recognised as an occupational disease of farmers who have worked with pesticides for more than 10 years[237]. Trichloroethylene is used in many detergents (degreasing and cleaning agents) and still widespread, even though several scientific studies have documented that people who have come into contact with such detergents have an ninefold risk of Parkinson's disease[238, 239]. Mould produces vapours containing octenol. Therefore, an individual's presence in mouldy rooms increases the risk of developing Parkinson's disease[240]. The massive poisoning of humanity with mercury from tooth amalgams, tuna, salmon and anchovies continues even though it is one of the most significant causes of Parkinson's disease. We refer to the chapter of this book: 'The influence of environmental stress from pollutants as the cause of neurogenerative diseases' (page 39). Patients suffering from diabetes mellitus more often develop Parkinson's disease later in life[241]. The number of years with the smoking habit increase the risk of Parkinson's disease more than the intensity of smoking[242, 243]. People with serious sleeping disorders or mental disorders have a higher risk of developing Parkinson's disease[244]. The neurodegenerative effect of pulsed high-frequency radiation together with scalar waves, as used in wireless telephony, is accumulative. This means that the risk of Parkinson's disease in later life increases proportionally to the number of minutes one spent phoning earlier in life[245]. The same applies to other neurodegenerative diseases and brain tumours. Because of the radiation pollution in buildings and towns, we can expect to see a massive increase of neurodegenerative diseases.

Nutrition and Parkinson's disease

Many epidemiological studies, as well as in vitro and in vivo examinations, have revealed a large number of factors that influence the risk of developing Parkinson's disease. These include general overeating, vitamins, flavonoids, selenium, coffee, alcohol, and the high content in saturated fatty acids in animal-based food and of toxic metals in fish products. Alcohol consumption and in particular beer considerably increases the risk of developing Parkinson's disease [246, 247, 248, 249]. Caffeine stimulates patients with Parkinson's disease and has a rather positive momentary effect on the motion disorder[250, 251]. However, nerve cells (neurons) protect from overload by discharging adenosine, which blocks the reception of nerve impulses by the neuron until it has recovered. Caffeine displaces adenosine from the receptors on the nerve cells and sabotages this natural protective mechanism. Although several studies have documented a protective effect of the caffeine in tea and coffee in relation to Parkinson's disease, we do not believe that patients with Parkinson's disease should consume caffeine-containing drinks over a long period (because of other detrimental effects of coffee as well). When meat is roasted, heterocyclic amines are produced as another important risk factor for neurodegenerative diseases[252]. Consuming alcohol considerably increases the risk for Parkinson's disease [253]. High urea levels result as a metabolic debt from a nutrition made up of large quantities of meat and dairy products. People with an increased urea level in the blood are at a higher risk of developing Parkinson's disease[254]. Because of decades using artificial fertilizers, many people are suffering from a selenium deficit today. Selenium protects against damage of the body's hereditary material from oxidative stress and heavy metals, and reduces lack of movement in artificially produced Parkinson's disease in animal studies[255]. An increased homocysteine level in the blood shows that not enough folic acid can be converted into its active form. This requires a generous supply of vitamin B_{12}. An increased homocysteine level is a sign of neurodegenerative diseases, such as Parkinson's disease. In contrast, high levels of folic acid, vitamin B_6 and B_{12} protect from this disease[256, 257]. Nutrition with little vitamin B_6, B_{12} or riboflavin increases the risk of Parkinson's disease[258]. Berries, in particular blue berries and eggplant/aubergine, contain the flavonoids antozian and proantozianidine, which are secondary plant substances that protect against Parkinson's disease by protecting the mitochondria from free radicals, thus protecting from the destruction of nerve cells in the substantia nigra and therefore against Parkinson's disease, even when a relatively low dose is involved[259, 260]. A low vitamin D level in the blood increase the risk of developing Parkinson's disease[261, 262]. Vegetable oils with polyunsaturated fatty acids, in particular omega-3 fatty acids, have an antioxidative and immunomodulating effect and protect from Parkinson's disease[263, 264, 265]. In an epidemiological study, Parkinson's disease was associated with high dairy consumption and with smoking. A high consumption of dairy products increases Parkinson risk in men[266]. The risk is lower in people who often consume polyunsaturated fatty acids[267]. An excessively high iron supply in the food (large quantities of meat), especially where there is high manganese content in the food, increases the risk of Parkinson's disease[268]. Overweight Parkinson patients are more likely to suffer from arrhythmia. This is explained by damage to the brain stem from α-synucleine deposits[269]. Nutrition with large quantities of animal-based fat (saturated fatty acids) increases the risk of developing Parkinson's disease [270, 271]. Overweight persons with type-II diabetes have a higher risk of Parkinson's disease, since the insulin resistance impairs the dopamine function in the nucleus niger[272, 235]. Reduction of the protein content in nutrition reduces Parkinson risk[273, 274, 275]. Increase of plant fibre in the nutrition improves the natural dopamine release in Parkinson's disease[276]. Nutrition with a high flavonoid content (with large quantities of fruit and vegetables) protects from Parkinson's disease[277]. A diet with a high content of vitamins E and β-carotene, which are contained in fruit, vegetables and unsaturated vegetable oils, reduces the risk of Parkinson's disease[278, 279]. Eliminating red meat from the diet and adding riboflavin improves movement in Parkinson's disease[280, 281]. A chronic iron deficit (reduced transferring saturation) is a risk factor for Parkinson's disease[282]. The consumption of fava beans increases the dopamine release of the neurons and thus particularly improves the movement disorder[283].

A Mediterranean diet contains large quantities of fruit, vegetables, vegetable oils and fish. It reduces the risk of Parkinson's disease[284, 285]. This is explained by the higher content of antioxidative plant-based food. Various cell cultures and animal models have shown that polyphenols and a diet rich in fruit and vegetables are effective against oxidative stress and thus not only protect from cancer and cardiovascular disease but also from neurodegenerative diseases such as Alzheimer's dementia and Parkinson's disease[286]. A Japanese case-control study with 368 patients showed an significant protective effect of nutrition consisting of large quantities of fruit, vegetables and fish against Parkinson's disease. (Note that the protective effect of the highly unsaturated fatty acids in fish oils can only be seen when eating them raw, since they are destroyed when cooking or roasting them[287].) There are indications that tomatoes protect from Parkinson's disease[288]. Today it is nutritionally and scientifically accepted that a diet with a high proportion of fruit and vegetables and rich in the amino acid S-adenosyl-L-methionine, vitamins B6, B12, C and folic acid in the food will protect from Alzheimer's dementia as well as Parkinson's disease[289]. In contrast, no protective effect was found when merely supplementing regular food with vitamins C and E at high dosages[290]. These antioxidants must be contained naturally in the food. A one-month study of 25 Parkinson patients compared 12 patients following a purely vegan diet with a control group of 13 patients following a normal, omnivorous diet. On the basis of the Parkinson rating scale, the Hoehn and Yahr Staging Scale and the Mann-Whitney test, the vegan group showed significant improvement in their ability to move, and a reduction in motion disturbances[291, 292].

The symptoms of Parkinson's disease

Parkinson's disease usually sets in between the ages of 50 and 79, and most often between the ages of 58 and 62. People older than 80 have a risk of slightly less than 2 %.

The disease starts slowly and usually on one side. One arm not swinging along when walking is an early sign. Often shoulder pain from muscle tension incites people to consult a doctor. Restricted movement (bradykinesia, akinesia) is decisive for diagnosis, with one of the three other principal symptoms: stiffness (rigor), characteristic trembling (tremor) and general insecurity when standing (postural instability)[293]. Restricted movement applies to all types of movement. The muscle capacity of facial expressions declines (mask-like face), and speech becomes slow and slurred. Swallowing is delayed and spittle becomes visible in front of the mouth. Fast movements of the hands become clumsy and writing becomes smaller. Movement becomes difficult so that the patients have trouble repositioning themselves in bed. Their gait develops into small steps and they drag their feet.

Rigidity and increased muscle tension causes muscle pain in patients. Limbs moved passively give way only with jerking rigidity (cogwheel phenomenon).

The trembling increases when the body is not in motion. Alternating tension of counteracting muscle groups at a slow rhythm of 4–9 beats per second appear, which makes the hands look as if one was turning something small between one's fingers ('pill-turning': 3 out of 4 patients with idiopathic Parkinson's syndrome display this, while it is rarer in atypical Parkinsonism).

All compensation reflexes when standing and walking are delayed, which makes standing and walking increasingly insecure. This is amplified by a heightened fear of falling.

The olfactory sense is also often reduced, and patients suffer from discomfort and from muscle and joint pain. Increased tallow volume production makes the face look glossy (salve face). The regulation of blood pressure is delayed, so that the patients risk losing consciousness and falling after getting up. Patients may also suffer from an excessively frequent urge to urinate (pollakisuria), from loss of libido, and from diarrhoea or obstipation. In the heat of summer, their ability to sweat is impaired, which may lead to potentially fatal overheating and or massive sweating at night. Patients often suffer from sleeping disorders and restless legs at night (restlessleg syndrome).

The mental effects of Parkinson's syndrome

Forty percent of Parkinson's patients suffer from melancholy moods. This often happens years before the other symptoms develop. Their thinking slows progressively (bradyphrenia), while their ability to think is maintained. A disturbance in the frontal brain leads to difficulties in estimating distances and speeds, which makes road traffic very dangerous for patients.

In addition, patients often suffer from hallucinations and anxieties that are a side effect of the dopaminergic medication[294, 295]. There are repeated lucid moments between the lack of motivation and lack of attention in which the remaining intelligence becomes obvious. However, the idiopathic form of Parkinson's disease will slowly lead to true dementia through the destruction of nerve cells by the LEWY-bodies. The mental changes cause great suffering. They are often underestimated because they are less obvious than the movement disorders.

Ensuring diagnosis of Parkinson's disease

Deposits of α-synucleine in the intestine and the salivary glands can be found in patients with Parkinson's disease. The levels of certain proteins in the brain fluid (liquor cerebrospinalis) are reduced and, as in Alzheimer's disease, TAU proteins

can be found with α-synuclein. To ensure the diagnosis, the loss of neurons in the substantia nigra can be documented reliably by single photon emission tomography after injecting iodine-123-FP-CIT or iodine-123-β-CIT[296]. MIBG-scintigraphy as used in heart diagnosis may be used to differentiate from multisystem atrophy (MSA). The severity of the dopamine deficit is determined with the L-Dopa test. A specific quantity of L-Dopa is indicated, and improvement in the ability to move is determined in the Unified Parkinson Disease Rating Scale (UPDRS). This proves only the degree of dopamine deficit, not the correct diagnosis of idiopathic Parkinson's disease. Similarly the apomorphine test is used for patients to whom L-Dopa cannot yet be administered
In the early stage of Parkinson's disease there will be a reduction of a number of proteins in the brain liquid in the spinal tap. There are also increased values for α-synucleins and TAU proteins, which are typical for Alzheimer's disease[297].

Atypical Parkinson's syndrome

These are severe neurodegenerative diseases in which degeneration occurs not only if the basal ganglia but also in other brain regions.

This includes rapidly progressing multisystem atrophy (MSA), where degeneration begins throughout the brain, corticobasal degeneration (CBD, LEWY-body dementia (LBD) and progressive supranuclear palsy (BSP, Steele-Richardson-Olszewski syndrome).

The treatment of Parkinson's disease

Pharmacological treatment
L-dopamine (Levodopa):
The most important anti-Parkinson remedy, L-dopamine (Levodopa) is a predecessor of dopamine, which penetrates the blood-brain barrier and is converted to dopamine in the brain. It replaces the missing dopamine. Since it only is effective for a few hours, there will often be unpleasant involuntary movements (dyskinesias) if used over several years, since the receptors are stimulated unevenly on account of the short time for which it is effective. Unfortunately this medicine loses its effectiveness over time, so that higher dosages and combinations will be necessary. Levodopa is always used in combination with a carboxylase inhibitor (Carbidopa, Benserazid), which inhibits the degradation of Levodopa before it enters the brain. Thus a lower dose of Levodopa and fewer side effects are possible for a longer period of time. There is no agreement on when Levodopa treatment should be begun. Whether waiting can delay the loss of efficacy is still open to debate. Levodopa is often used as soon as the patient is impaired in his everyday life in spite of amantadine or anticholinergic substances. Meals high in protein may lead to temporary deterioration (fluctuation). It is suspected that certain amino acids conflict with the intake of L-Dopa at the blood-brain barrier, resulting in lower efficacy[298]. A low-protein diet improves the movement disorder in Parkinson's disease[299].

Dopamine agonists:
This category includes the traditional ergot alkaloids (Bromocriptin, Cabergolin, Dihydroergocryptin, Lisurid, Pergulid). They imitate the effect of dopamine. In younger patients especially treatment is started with these substances to avoid dyskinesias (movement disorders). Today there are medicines that do not act to the same extent on the entire body, but more selectively on the dopamine receptors. They are called D2-receptor agonists or non-ergot dopamine agonists (Apomorphin, Pribedil, Pramipexol, Ropinirol, Rotigotin, Bromocriptin). They

differ in their effective duration and their side effects.

Amantadine:
Originally developed against viruses, they increase the dopamine content in the synaptic gap. Higher dopamine content mainly counters the lack of movement (akinesia). Over time the skin will turn blue (cyanosis) and water will be deposited in it (oedema).

MAO-inhibitors (Selegilin, Rasagilin):
They inhibit the degradation of dopamine by inhibiting the enzyme monoamin-oxidase that causes degradation.

Anticholinergic substances (Biperidin, Trihexiphenyl):
The deficit of dopamine causes the antagonist acetyl choline to be predominant in Parkinsonism. They mostly act to combat 'excess symptoms', trembling (tremor) and rigidity (rigor). However, because they impair mental performance, they are now used almost exclusively to treat Parkinsonism, which is induced by psychiatric medication (neuroleptics).

COMT-inhibitors (Catechol-0-Methyl-transferase inhibitors):
Medicines (Entacarpon, Tolcapon) inhibit the degradation of the dopamine precursors and are only used in combination with L-Dopa and in combination with a decarboxylase inhibitor (Carbidopa or Benserazid), thereby lowering the doses of Levodopa and reducing its side effects. The decarboxylase inhibitors reduce the concentration of COMT inhibitors in the body and thus the side effects. They increase the availability of the Levodopa which is taken at the same time by 40–90 %. Because Entacarpon can severely damage the liver, liver values must be monitored frequently.

Vegetable L-dopamine:
Mucuna pruriens contains the dopamine precursor L-dopamine and therefore is effective. Since the content of Levodopa is neither standardised nor stable, adjustment of the effect is usually unsatisfactory. This is due to its varging concentration in the brain, that leads to fluctuations, an effect which causes the degree of the movement disorder to fluctuate excessively.

Neurosurgical treatment
Brainstem stimulation:
This method, used when medicines prove inadequate, requires a programmable brain pacemaker, which conducts impulses to the affected brainstem ganglia by means of thin wires. This is to enable patients to continue to drive unassisted[300]. However, placement of the electrodes in the brain takes 8–9 hours; it is difficult and harmful to the patient and does not always improve symptoms. This intervention often leads to a speech disorder (dysarthria) and an unpleasant increase in the drive to be active, which is usually limited to one year.

Gene therapy
In this treatment, genetically engineered viruses (the corpus striatum of the brain) are implanted in the brain, where they should improve enzyme activity so that more dopamine is provided.

Implantation of foetal brain tissue
Trials with the implementation of embryonic stem cells for nerve tissue unfortunately have not yet lead to satisfactory results.

Comprehensive treatment for Parkinson's disease

Immediate elimination of the causes is critical for progress to be made. Elimination includes careful diagnosis and the discharge from the body of toxic metals; diagnosis regarding neurotoxic contamination at home and at work, diagnosis of the electromagnetic and empathic stress in the bedroom, in all locations where the patient spends time, and at the workplace. Such stress must be removed immediately and as thoroughly as possible.

Patients with Parkinson's disease usually suffer from severe oxidative stress that can be diagnosed and eliminated through a low-protein, vegetarian fresh food diet with a high proportion of raw food, a high content of polyunsaturated fatty acids in a therapeutically suitable ratio (the same amount of omega-6 and omega-3 in vegetable oil, antioxidative vitamins and phytochemicals). We also conduct a high-dosage antioxidative infusion treatment with glutathione, vitamin C, alpha liponic acid and amino acids that act on the brain metabolism, as well as ubiquinone (coenzyme Q10). The folic acid, vitamin B_6, B_{12} and vitamin D levels must be taken to the upper norm. These measures often delay the need for medication and allow for much lower doses with fewer side effects. Unfortunately no studies have been carried out with regard to this treatment. We have to base our explanations on our decades of experience, which have shown that this treatment can significantly influence the disease's progress.

The commencement of Parkinson symptoms raises questions about the meaning of life and the natural limitation of life that affects us all. Questions are also raised about the meaning of our relationships and the meaning of the disease for the patient personally. There remain many tactics that we can employ to rid ourselves of whatever was senseless in life in order to liberate ourselves from insults, enmities, envy and supposed riches. The goal is to align ourselves with something new, something more essential, with inner values and renewed humanity: a new inner wealth that enables us to better understand and help others and ourselves.

The dietary treatment corresponds to that which is effective for all neurodegenerative diseases and is explained and described below for simple, practical use.

Dietary treatment of neurodegenerative diseases

Fresh, plant-based food (raw vegetarian food) is decisive for successful treatment because of the very order of its energy potential that can regenerate cells. The "information" from sunlight that is absorbed through photosynthesis renews the LASER amplification in the genetic material, the DNA of the cells, so that its energy is and remains removed from the thermodynamic balance so that the second main principle of thermodynamics does not apply. The ordering, regenerating principle (Prigogine's coherence principle) prevails over Clausius' degenerating chaos principle.

A high proportion of fruit and vegetables in the diet is the most effective protection against degenerative conditions[301]. The recommendations of the Deutsche Gesellschaft für Ernährung (DGE) have been adapted as a consequence of this insight[301]. Note Bircher-Benner manual no. 4: Fresh juices, raw vegetables and fruit dishes, and Bircher-Benner manual no. 24: For the prevention of dementia and Alzheimer's disease.

The high content of pharmacologically active substances in raw food, the secondary plant substances (phytochemicals), and specifically those with antioxidative effects, are also very important. We have seen how much the oxidative stress from toxins, high-frequency radiation and an unhealthy lifestyle and nutrition contrary to the needs of our biological nature are the root cause of the harmful effects on the nerve cells (neurons) described above. The diet should have a very high antioxidative potential that is capable of capturing and neutrlizing free radicals. Every vegetarian raw food dish has a high antioxidative potential if the plant from which it is derived is capable of performing photosynthesis. Plants with particularly strong antioxidative (and therefore regenerative) effects should be preferred. These are foods with a high content of flavonoids and carotenoids. Flavonoids are found in particular in the outer layers of fruits and vegetables. Therefore they are mostly lost when vegetables and fruits are peeled. The protective effect of the carotenoids (xanthines), however, is lost in cooking[302].

Carotenoids
These are the red and yellow pigments in fruits, roots, leaves and vegetables. They fight cancer, modulate the immune system and achieve an antioxidative effect by neutralising free radicals. Free radicals are highly reactive disintegration products of the water or nitrogen-oxygen molecules that mutate healthy cells into cancer cells.

Oxygen-containing carotenoids are lutein, zeaxanthin and β-cryptoxanthin. They mostly occur in the yellow and red parts of plants and are relatively stable in heat, so that they remain effective when cooked. Lutein is particularly important for the retina in the eye, the cells of which are specialised nerve cells of the brain. Oxygen-free carotenoids are lycopene, α-carotene and ß-carotene. They occur mostly in the green parts of plants and are sensitive to heat. Therefore an essential part of the antioxidative effect of carotenoids that protects from cancer is lost when cooking green vegetables. Raw carrots and pumpkins are particularly rich in α-carotene. Apricots, green cabbage, spinach, pumpkins and carrots are particularly rich in β-carotene when not heated. Lycopene is found almost exclusively in tomatoes. Lutein and zeaxanthin, which are important for the retina, are found mainly in green cabbage and spinach, where cooking only destroys them very slightly. About 10 % of the carotenoids act as provitamin A, which is converted into the antioxidative active vitamin A.

Flavonoids
Flavonoids have an antioxidative effect. They are found in the outer layers of fruits and vegetables, but also in their leaves. Yellow flavonoids, as contained in yellow fruits and vegetables, have given these substances their name (*flavus* means 'yellow'). The flavonoid group of anthrozians provides the red, yellow and violet colours, as in cherries, plums, berries, red cabbage and aubergines. The flavonoid quercetin is very common. Its glycoside (quercetin bound to sugar) is called rutine. Quercetin is common in yellow onions and (in descending order) green cabbage, green beans, apples, cherries and broccoli. Quercetin is metabolised by the intestinal flora. It destroys carcinogenic substances (carcinogens)[302].

Flavonoids are highly effective antioxidants. In addition, they are active against pathogens and cancer. Their ability to modulate the disturbed immune system concomitant with neurodegenerative diseases, as well as their anti-inflammatory effect in the cerebral immune system of the microglia, which maintains the destructive processes in the nervous system, are essential for preventing and healing such conditions. Flavonoids also regulate the permeability of the capillary blood vessels (vascular permeability)[301]. They supplement the effects of vitamin C.

Although flavonoids are not destroyed by cooking, they can be destroyed by storage. Stored winter apples contain 50 % of their flavonoids. In August, head lettuce and endives contain five times as many flavonoids as in April. Processed foods have about 50 % of the flavonoid content of freshly harvested fruits[303].

Polyphenols
These substances (phenols, phenolic acids, cumarins, flavonoids, isoflavonoids, lignans, lignins, etc.) are highly active antioxidants. They protect the outer layers of the plant, and thus its inner parts, against oxidation. Green cabbage, whole wheat grains, radishes and white cabbage are particularly rich in polyphenols, followed by green and other fruits, nuts and coffee beans. Carrots contain 85 % of their polyphenols in their skin, and wheat has the largest share in the bran. Wholemeal wheat contains 10 times more polyphenols than coarsely ground wheat flour. When stored, the polyphenols are gradually oxidised and lose their effect. If parts of a plant turn brown or black, the polyphenols are converted into toxic chinons by the enzyme phenoloxidase. Such parts are toxic and must not be eaten. The polyphenol ellagic acid induces (activates) detoxing enzymes in the intestinal mucosa (phase II enzymes) and thus reduces carcinogenic substances. Walnuts are particularly rich in ellagic acid, followed by fresh blackberries and raspberries, strawberries and pecan nuts. When cooking jam, three-quarters of the polyphenols in the berries are lost. Polyphenols are metabolised very quickly. Therefore fresh fruits, nuts and raw vegetables provide protection only if eaten several times a day, i.e. at each meal.

Protease inhibitors
These secondary plant substances split up proteins into amino acids. The protease inhibitors of the plants are chains of approx. 100 amino acids that are connected by disulphide bridges (sulphur bridges). Protease inhibitors not only protect from

cancer and diabetes, they also have an antioxidative and anti-inflammatory effect and thus counter degenerative processes. They are also very important for the prevention of and fight against neurodegenerative processes.

Protease inhibitors are contained in fresh soy beans, mung beans, garden peas, unroasted peanuts, potatoes, rice, corn, oats and wheat. They are shown to have an anti-carcinogenic effect in animal studies[304].

Terpens
These are aromatics (smell and taste substances) of plants. The terpen limonene of lemons increases the activity of detoxification enzymes in the small intestine and the liver, including Glutathione-S-transferase. Limonene and carvon from caraway are effective for combatting cancer[305] in animal experiments. Limonene, derived from the essential oil of lemons, is not toxic even at high doses. Therefore it is particularly suitable for fighting neurodegeneration and cancer.

Sulphides
The sulphur compounds of the sulphides are what give onion and garlic their typical smell. The volatile (pungent smelling) garlic oil consists of different allyl sulphides. The main effect of garlic is caused by allicin, its characteristic aromatic substance. Allicin has a strong protective effect against oxidation and against the effect of free radicals. This makes it particularly valuable for the prevention of and fight against neurodegenerative conditions.

Vitamins A, C, D, E, folic acid and polyunsaturated vegetable oils
As we have seen, the blood levels of vitamins A, C, D and E are very important for the prevention and healing of neurodegenerative processes. Vegetarian fresh food is very rich in folic acid.

Vitamin B_{12} is highly relevant for the conversion of the precursors of folic acid into its active form. Plant-based vitamin B_{12} is only found in hawthorn. It can be difficult to find fresh. It can be taken every day as an unsweetened elixir. Nevertheless the vitamin B_{12} level must be monitored at regular intervals and restored to the upper standard limit, with suitable preparations if necessary. Vitamins D and E are contained in cold-pressed vegetable oils such as sunflower oil, sunflowerr oil, rapeseed oil, sesame oil, walnut oil, flaxseed oil, etc.
The polyunsaturated vegetable oils (PUFA) omega-3 and omega-6 act upon the immune system. Therefore it is very important to observe their ratios, since the ratio of omega-3 to omega-6 is often too low. Omega-6 vegetable oils have an antioxidative effect but stimulate inflammation processes, while omega-3 vegetable oils also have a strongly antioxidative effect but dampen the immune system. We have seen that excessive inflammatory processes in neurodegenerative diseases are very significant in relation to the degeneration of the nervous system. Therefore we recommend taking three tablespoons of flaxseed oil three times a day in any case. We have already explained why fish oils should no longer be used to supply omega-3 oils. Vitamin D is assimilated better when taken together with flaxseed oil.

A raw food vegetarian diet is very rich in vitamin C with its high bioavailability. The vitamin D level should be brought to the upper standard level through regular exposure to the sun (20 minutes per body side without sun blocker, but with the head covered, and not during the three hottest hours) and if necessary by taking suitable vitamin D preparations.

The intestinal flora and the enteral immune system

The effect of raw food for the restoration of the milieu in the gastrointestinal tract is very important. We have seen that the immune cells learn to acquire their immune competence, in the lymph cell nests of the intestinal mucosa (Payer's plaques) and to differentiate foreign, toxic, harmful substances and germs from the body's own useful and beneficial substances and germs; and that subsequently only approx. 10 % of them will migrate into the body as immunocompetent cells to assume their tasks there.

In all neurodegenerative diseases, but especially multiple sclerosis, autoimmune processes are closely involved in the destruction of the nervous system. Vegetarian food – especially when as fresh as possible – restores the milieu in the gastrointestinal tract in a relatively rapid and thorough manner. A vegetarian diet high in fresh raw food slowly replaces with aerobic, healthy intestinal bacteria the germs growing anaerobically that produce putrefaction toxins and that have developed in an environment of high-protein nutrition. The miscolonisation reduces and disappears entirely within a few months. Now immunocompetent lymph cells are developed again. This reliably reduces the autoimmune processes and finally brings them to a complete halt, so that the inflammatory processes in the nervous system subside. Refer to the Bircher-Benner manual no. 14: For patients with gastrointestinal conditions.

Lab control recommendations for the attending physician during the diet

Before beginning the diet: complete blood count, ESR, CRP, homocysteine, Na, K, selenium, zinc, serum-albumin, GOT, GPT, pancreas amylase, LDH, vitamins A, D and B_{12}, TSH. We recommend regularly monitoring the levels of vitamins B_{12} and D and consistently replacing them to the upper standard level during the treatment.

Table on the effects of foods on neurodegenerative diseases

	Antioxidative and antidegenerative effect	Inhibition of inflammation	Immunomodulation
Apple	+++u	++u	+++u
Apricot	+++	++	++r+
Aubergine	+++	++	++
Avocado	+++		++
Berry	+++	++	+++
Pear	++	++u	+++u
Blueberry	+++	++	++++*
Leafy salad	+++		++
Fennel	++	++	++
Pomegranate	+++	+++	++
Grapefruit	+++	+++	+++
Cucumber	+++	++	++
Legume	++		++++
Carrot	+++++	++u	+++++u, raw
Potato	++	++raw, m	++
Chickpea			
Kiwi	+++	++	+++
Bran	+++		
Garlic	+++++raw	+++++raw	+++++raw
Cabbage	++++	++	++
Coconut	++++	++	++
Cress	+++		
Pumpkin	+++		
Lettuce	+++	++	+++
Leek	++		
Flaxseed oil, Flaxseed raw	+++++++lip	+++++lip	+++++lip
Lychee	+++	++	+++
Corn	+		
Mango	+++	++	
Horseradish raw	++	++	++
Melon	+++	+++	+++
Nut	++		++++
Papaya	+++	++	+++
Pepper	+++	++	+++
Passion fruit	+++	++	+++

	Antioxidative and antidegenerative effect	Inhibition of inflammation	Immunomodulation
Plant oil, polyunsaturated (PUFA)	+++++	[lip]	+++++[lip]
Radish types	++++		+++
Beetroot	+++	++	+++
Celery (celeriac)	++		+++
Soy	++[raw]		++++[raw]
Spinach	+++[raw]		++
Stone fruit	++++	++	+++
Grape	+++	++	+++
Tomato	+++[raw]	++[raw]	+++ [raw]
Whole cereal	++		++[raw]
Citrus fruit	+++		+++
Onion	+++[raw]	++++ [raw]	++++ [raw]

u: The polyphenols are in the skins of fruit and vegetables, which therefore should not be peeled. Approx. 50 % of the benefits are lost when fruit and vegetables are stored.

lip: Oils with polyunsaturated fatty acids (PUFA) e.g. flaxseed, sunflower, sesame, nut, sunflower, rapeseed, grapeseed, etc., must never be heated. Flaxseed oil must be stored in a cool, dark place. Olive oil contains mostly monounsaturated fatty acids and therefore may be heated to 170° C. Flaxseed oil moderates the immune system and therefore counters inflammation. A 1:1 ratio of omega-6 oil to omega-3 oil is the target for dietary treatment of neurodegenerative diseases.

Table on the general effect of raw food therapy

This table shows general indications and effects that can be considered in treatment:

Preparation	Treatment	Effect	Duration	Quantity
Juice: fruit, raw vegetables, plant milk (almond soy, sesame) certified raw milk, if prescribed: additions of whole cereal or flaxseed gruel (always ⅓ of the juice) or cream and a little lemon juice	general metabolism overload (fasting indication), obesity, heart and circulatory failure, gastrointestinal inflammation, kidney and liver inflammations, acute flu (fever)	detoxifying, relieving, dehydrating (relieves heart and circulation), seals vessels, reduces inflammation, deacidifying, promotes nutritional economy, restores the intestinal milieu, reduces weight	1 – 28 days depending on medical prescription 1 – 3 days for longer fasting treatments	600 – 800 g fresh juices (3 – 4 glasses) 450 – 500 g plant milk or herbal tea 200 – 400 calories

Preparation	Treatment	Effect	Duration	Quantity
Pureed (slightly greater quantity, oil added): fruit and vegetables mixed in the blender (vegetables with sauce, see recipes), plant milk (almond, soy, sesame), certified raw milk, sour milk, butter milk, whey, yoghurt	inflammations in the digestive system, convalescence	same as under 'juice', plus cellulose content (stimulation of the peristaltic), addition of oil	3–14 days depending on medical prescription	approx. 1200 calories (see daily menu)
Finely chopped: fruit and vegetables, finely cut, chopped (for sauces, see the recipe section) walnuts, almonds, hazelnuts finely ground; addition: plant or raw certified raw milk, buttermilk, sour milk, whey, yoghurt wholemeal grain: finely chopped or sprouted	as under 'pureed' further convalescence	as under 'pureed': fermentative peristaltic effect by cellulose in coarser form, more volume, higher saturation form, stimulation of the intestine	3–21 days depending on medical prescription	800–1200 calories; see daily menu
Normal raw vegetables: fruit and vegetables whole or chopped (Bircher muesli) normally prepared (see recipe section) walnuts, almonds, hazelnuts, pine nuts (whole). Whole cereal: chopped, coarsely ground or in flakes. Certified raw milk, raw buttermilk and sour milk, whey, yoghurt	general realignment of the metabolic reaction obstipation eczema and any allergic diseases, migraine acne, furunculosis, chron. infection and susceptibility to infection, arteriosclerosis, hypertension, preparation and aftertreatment of surgery, rheumatism	can be applied for weeks and months, forces increased chewing as a coarser form and stimulates the saliva glands, mechanical cleaning of the teeth	on average 1–6 weeks or 1–3 days per week alternating with juice fasting, raw food with additions (see p. 94)	1200–1700 calories; see daily menu

Practical application of the raw food therapy

When there is no question of kidney failure, it is usually best to begin the diet with the first diet level (the fresh juice and plant milk diet), since this will convert the metabolism and intestinal milieu the fastest. The patient will not feel hungry. See Bircher-Benner manual no. 4: On fresh juices, raw vegetables and fruit dishes, which should be read before starting the diet. After a patient-specific duration, it can be replaced by the second diet level (the vegan raw food diet). After the disease has developed, this diet form is the most effective. It can and should be continued for many weeks or months. Later the third diet level can be used, e.g. on weekends, with one-third hot meals. A cyclical approach has also proven to be valuable, e.g. using level I on Monday, level II during the week and level III on the weekends. The following menus and recipe suggestions have proven their worth for decades and have been designed in accordance with this procedure.

Menus

Menus for various raw food regimes

1. Fresh juice fasting (bed/juice day)
Morning and evening: 200 g fruit juice
Lunch: 200 g fruit juice or
200 g vegetable juice (tomato or carrot juice, or a mix of tomato, carrot and spinach juice)
Depending on the season:
orange and tangerine juice
grapefruit juice
berry juices
grape juice
plum juice
peach juice
apricot juice,
Japanese persimmon (kaki) juice
apple and pear juice (fresh)

These juices can also be combined (e.g. berry with peach or apricot juice, apricot with orange juice, apple with pear juice).

Depending on doctor's orders, fresh juice fasting may be undertaken for one or several days – even two, three or (rarely) four weeks. Medical supervision during fasting and subsequent recuperation is important (see table on page 91). If only mild effects of fasting are desired – in the sense of general detoxification, dehydration and rejuvenation – a strict fruit juice day can be used once a week within the raw food treatment or regular diet where complete rest (preferably bed rest) is possible. If you do not rest during the first one or two fasting days, the full effect will be impaired by fatigue and hunger, and there will not be proper relaxation and urine flow. Do not be deterred by reactions such as headache, nausea, pain in the limbs, and weakness (especially in the afternoon). These show that the body is doing its detoxification work during juice fasting, so that such days have meaning and purpose. Be sure to report your observations to your doctor.

2. Juice only day
High quality, relatively nutritious food is administered. This regime can be maintained for one week or longer with the addition of cereal gruels, and can be prolonged for several weeks with the avoidance of strong physical and mental stress. Juice only periods are suitable to start readjustment treatment, for dewatering and weight loss treatments or, if the organism is very low in respect of vital substance (e.g. in the case of chronic digestive diseases if a traditional bland raw food free diet has been administered). In such cases, fruit juice should initially be taken with ⅓ flaxseed, barley or rice gruel. For dehydration treatments, urine and weight must be measured at regular intervals. If necessary, diuretic tea (solidago, rosehip) should be drunk.

Morning: 200 g fruit juice
150 g almond milk or yoghurt
1 cup of rosehip tea
Lunch: 200 g fruit juice
150 g almond milk or yoghurt
150 g vegetable juice

Evening: same as morning.

3. Fruit fasting days
Fruit fasting may replace juice fasting in bed (the strict form of the fruit juice fasting day), e.g. when metabolism change

and stimulation of the intestine with cellulose content is the principal aim, rather than protection through free cellulose. Since this diet produces a strong feeling of satiation, fruit fasting can be performed even on days without complete rest, and for extended periods of time. However, the effect of juice fasting is more intense. Fruit fasting is indicated for persons with heart disease, chronic liver weakness, or lazy bowels. Other indications are an apple day for acute diarrhea and a strawberry day for celiac disease and abdominal congestion. Duration: 1–5 days (longer if prescribed by the doctor).

Daily menu: 3 times 200–250 g (up to 300 g) washed, fresh, completely ripe, unsweetened fruit, e.g. berries, citrus fruit (oranges, grapefruit, tangerines), grapes, figs, melons, Japanese persimmons (kaki).

Special fruit fasting forms
Apple day: 5–6 times 1 large apple finely grated for acute gastrointestinal catarrh with diarrhoea.

Strawberry day: 3–4 times 200–250 g very ripe strawberries, unsweetened, for celiac disease (special form of chronic diarrhoea) and vitamin C deficit.

Blueberry day: 3 times 200–250 g blueberries for slight intestinal infection. Slightly constipating.

Blackberry day: 3 times 200–250 g completely ripe blackberries. Particularly rich in natural sugar and vitamin C. Nutritious and easy to digest.

Currant day: 3 times 200–250 g (⅔ red and yellow, ⅓ black). For patients with liver problems particularly refreshing and thirst-relieving. Rich in vitamin C.

Japanese persimmon (kaki) day: 2 small (or 1 large) Japanese persimmon fruits, 4 times a day. Very nutritious and rich in vitamins C and B.

Grape day (traditional grape treatment): 750–1000 g sun-ripened grapes, organically grown, distributed over 4–5 meals per day. Wash thoroughly and remove any treatment residue (briefly wash in hot water). Eat whole fruit. Low in vitamins but particularly nutritious because of its high fruit sugar content. Liver protection. Stimulates intestine with seeds. Duration: 1–2 weeks, longer if prescribed by doctor (up to 6 weeks).

Fig day: 3 times 200 g fresh figs. Stimulates the intestine. Nutritious. No more than 1 day.

4. Raw Vegetable Menus
Below are seven examples of raw vegetable combinations for lunch for each season. (Special value is placed on the harmonious distribution of bulb, root and leaf raw vegetables, but always use them fresh and very ripe). For a full daily menu, see page 96.

a) Spring:
1st day: fruits – nuts (also dried fruit) – radishes – fennel – head lettuce
2nd day: fruits – nuts – celery root (celeriac) – tomatoes – cress
3rs day: fruits – nuts – carrots – chicory/endive – head lettuce
4th day: fruits – nuts – radish – lettuce – cress
5th day: fruits – nuts – beetroot – dandelion – head lettuce
6th day: fruits – nuts – cauliflower – spinach – cress
7th day: fruits – nuts – kohlrabi – tomatoes – head lettuce

b) Summer:
1st day: fruits – nuts – radish – tomatoes – head lettuce
2nd day: fruits – nuts – carrots – courgettes – head lettuce

3rd day: fruits – nuts – cauliflower – radishes – head lettuce
4th day: fruits – nuts – kohlrabi – cress – head lettuce
5th day: fruits – nuts – celery root (celeriac) – lettuce – head lettuce
6th day: fruits – nuts – tomatoes stuffed with cauliflower – head lettuce
7th day: fruits – nuts – small carrots – cucumbers – head lettuce

c) Autumn:
1st day: fruits – nuts – celery root (celeriac) – tomatoes – endives/chicory
2nd day: fruits – nuts – beetroot – peppers – head lettuce
3rd day: fruits – nuts – black salsify – spinach – head lettuce
4th day: fruits – nuts – cauliflower – lamb's lettuce – endives
5th day: fruits – nuts – small carrots – courgettes – cress
6th day: fruits – nuts – radish – tomatoes – head lettuce
7th day: fruits – nuts – celery root (celeriac) – cucumbers – head lettuce

d) Winter:
1st day: fruits – nuts – black salsify – red cabbage – endives
2nd day: fruits – nuts – celery root (celeriac) – radicchio – head lettuce
3rd day: fruits – nuts – carrots – sweet pepper – head lettuce
4th day: fruits – nuts – beetroot – sauerkraut – endives/chicory
5th day: fruits – nuts – cauliflower – spinach – lamb's lettuce
6th day: fruits – nuts – tomatoes – chicory/endive – head lettuce
7th day: fruits – nuts – celery root (celeriac) – Savoy cabbage – chicory/endive

Daily menu

Breakfast

Bircher muesli	120–200 g
Ground almonds or hazelnuts	20–30 g
Fruits	100–200 g
Optional rosehip tea	1 cup

If a mushy or liquid consistency is desired: Bircher muesli with finely ground or mixed fruits (with cream, optional, 100–200 g), almond milk (20–30 g almond puree), 150 g fruit juice and 1 cup of rosehip tea. The quantities need only approximate to those indicated. What is important is the natural feeling that must not be impaired by stimulants or habits. Only where very little nutrition is desired should hunger be reduced by long chewing and salivation and by a slower intake of food.

Lunch

Fruits or chilled fruit soup	150–250 g
Green lettuce	50–100 g
Raw vegetable plate	approx. 100–150 g
Nuts of all kinds	approx. 20 g
1 glass of unfermented apple or grape juice (optional)	200 g

or

Fruit juice	approx. 100–200 g
Green lettuce, finely chopped	approx. 50 g
Raw vegetables blended or mashed (cucumbers, tomatoes)	100 g
Vegetable juice (spinach, carrots, etc.) with a touch of cream and lemon juice	100 g
Almond milk or sesame milk	approx. 200 g
Optional apple or grape juice	200 g

Dinner

Bircher muesli	150–200 g
Nuts	20–30 g
Fruits	100–200 g
Optional rosehip tea	1 cup

Or

Bircher muesli	150–200 g
Almond milk	approx. 200 g
Fruit juice	approx. 200 g
Optional rosehip tea	1 cup

5. Temporary and regular food
When patients have not relapsed for at least one year, they can add one third cooked food to their raw food diet, starting out entirely vegan. After two years they may carefully and sparingly add dairy products and eggs. It is important that they use raw food phases in between at regular intervals.

In the chapter 'Recipes', foods that are not vegan are marked with a *.

Example for a temporary day
Morning and evening: Same as raw food day.

Lunch: Fruits, nuts, raw vegetable plate, 2 dl vegetable bouillon
2 baked potatoes (see recipe page 115)

Example for a normal diet day
Breakfast:
Bircher muesli with ground nuts, 2 slices of wholemeal bread or crispbread, approx. 15 g butter (optional)
Fruits
Herbal tea, or milk or yoghurt

Lunch:
Fruits
Raw vegetables: cauliflower, spinach, head lettuce
Potato soup
Steamed tomato, vegetables
Whole rice with fresh butter only, no cheese, lightly salted

Dinner:
Same as breakfast, optional rosehip jam or honey as bread spread.

The Recipes

Recipes marked * are not vegan. They must only be used in the menu plan after two years without a relapse. Individual non-vegan ingredients that can be left out or replaced are also marked with an *.

Juices

Juices are from raw fruits and vegetables in a mechanically refined form, used as additional special enrichment, when coarse food (cellulose) is not permitted. Whole raw vegetables are always higher in their nutritional quality and cannot be permanently replaced by juice.

For the preparation of juices, raw vegetables must be cleaned thoroughly, pressed with a hand press or an electric centrifugal juicer, and served immediately. Letting them stand reduces their value.

If a small hand press is used, fruits and vegetables must be chopped. Grate apples, pears and all bulbous vegetables finely; chop leafy vegetables and herbs finely.

High quality grape, fruit and vegetable juices are available at health food stores.

Fruit juices
Unmixed fruit juices (without any additives)
Orange, tangerine, grapefruit, apple, pear, grape, strawberry, blueberry, currant, cassis, raspberry, peach, apricot, plum, mango, Japanese persimmon (kaki), kiwi.

Mixed fruit juices
For example orange, tangerine, grapefruit, Japanese persimmon (kaki) or berry juice with apple juice or berry juice with peach, apricot or plum juice or whipped bananas with orange, berry, peach, mango or apricot juice.

Additions to taste or as needed: lemon juice, honey, maple syrup, fruit concentrate, cream, yoghurt, almond milk (only to be used if patient also suffers from stomach complaints), flaxseed, rice or barley gruel.

Vegetable juices
When fresh they have a high mineral and vitamin content. Each juice has its own special value.

Unmixed vegetable juices
Tomato, carrot, beetroot, radish, cabbage, celery root (celeriac), potatoes, all leaf, bulbous and root vegetables; stinging nettle, sorrel and dandelion juice for springtime blood-cleansing treatment.

Mixed vegetable juices
Carrot, tomato, and spinach in equal proportions (very good flavour)
tomato and carrot
tomato and spinach.
Other mixes (and cocktails) can be combined according to taste.
For variety, add sorrel, stinging nettle, chives, parsley, onions, tender celery leaves or roots, and other herbs.
Additions per glass (1½–2 dl): a little lemon juice, fruit concentrate (optional, small quantity). Flaxseed (optional), rice or barley gruel. Other leafy vegetables or

lettuces may be used, such as white cabbage, endives/chicory, lamb's lettuce, lettuce, dandelion.

Potato juice
Prepare scrubbed, peeled (optional) potatoes (do not use potatoes that are unripe, green or sprouted) as for carrot juice. Not very agreeable and only to be used on doctor's orders.

Gruel to accompany juices
The gruel is added to raw juices in a proportion of 1:3 it neutralises the sharpness of the fruit or vegetable flavour. Only to be used if the patient also suffers from stomach complaints. The daily ration can be prepared once a day and kept cool in a thermos flask.

Rice or barley gruel
Stir 1 heaped teaspoon of rice or barley wholemeal flour with 2 dl cold water and boil for 5 minutes, stirring constantly. Let cool.

Flaxseed gruel
Rinse 1 tablespoon flaxseeds, boil in 2 dl water for 10 minutes, strain and let cool.

Bircher muesli

All recipes are for 1 person.

Bircher muesli
In our long experience, the original apple muesli as invented by Dr Bircher and used successfully thousands of times with his patients has remained the best food for the regime.

Sweet-tart juicy apples with white flesh are best for muesli (e.g. Klar, Gravenstein, Sauergrauech, Menznauer Jäger, Jonathan, Ontario, Rubinette, Glockenäpfel, Braeburn, Topas, Champagner-Reinetten, Cox's Orange, Gala).

The flavour of drier apple types with a blander taste can be enriched with a pinch of the freshly grated peel of untreated oranges or lemons, or with orange juice, a little rosehip paste or freshly grated ginger.

Bircher muesli with yoghurt, sour milk or buttermilk*
1 tbs oat flakes
3 tsp water
1 tbs lemon juice
2 tsp Bifidus yoghurt, Bifidus sour milk or buttermilk
1 tsp honey
200 g apples
1 tbs hazelnuts or almonds, ground

Soak the oat flakes for 12 hours (overnight if for breakfast). Mix the oat flakes, yoghurt (or sour milk) and honey until smooth. Remove stems and calyxes from the washed apples and, using the Bircher grater, grate the apples into the sauce. Stir several times to keep the muesli attractively white. Spread the nuts on it and serve at once.

Other versions: Replace oat flakes with wheat, rice, barley, rye, semolina, buckwheat or soy flakes, optionally mixed with yeast flakes (enriching the muesli with vitamin B).

Different version: Mix 1 teaspoon soaked oat flakes with 1 teaspoon cereal grains (Soak in water for 24 hrs., then put through a sieve and rinse with cold water.) Whole, chopped or mixed.

Bircher muesli with almond or sesame puree (vegan) (basic recipe)
1 tbs oat flakes
3 tsp water
½ tbs lemon juice
1 tbs almond or sesame puree
1 tsp honey
3 tsp water
200 g apples
1 tbs hazelnuts or almonds, ground

Soak oat flakes for 12 hours. Stir in lemon juice, puree, honey and water with a whisk to produce a creamy consistency, add the oat flakes and apples (prepared like basic recipe). Spread the nuts on top and serve at once.

Bircher muesli with cream*
(Specially enriched recipe designed for weight gain.) For diabetics, no honey or oat flakes. For diabetics with a low-fat diet, with unsugared condensed milk.
1 tbs (8 g) fine oat flakes
3 tsp water
½ tsp lemon juice 3–4 tsp cream
1 tbs honey
200 g apples
1 tbs hazelnuts or almonds, ground

Prepared as for basic recipe.

Bircher muesli with berries or stone fruit
Rich in vitamin C.
Prepare an almond puree, sesame puree or yoghurt sauce.
Add
150–200 g strawberries or raspberries, blueberries, currants or blackberries, and mash slightly with a fork.
Or
150–200 g plums, peaches or apricots, pitted and passed through the chopper or cut finely with a knife.

Bircher muesli with various fruits
The following combinations are very tasty:

strawberries and raspberries,
strawberries and currants
strawberries and apples blackberries and apples
apples with finely cut orange and tangerine segments
apples and bananas
apples and peaches
sauce: almond or sesame puree sauce, or yoghurt sauce

Use only fresh fruits, never use canned fruits (fruit salad, etc.).

Bircher muesli with dried fruits
If you have no fresh fruits at hand, you can also make the muesli with dried fruits (apples, apricots, plums, pears). One hundred grammes of dried fruits are washed, soaked in cold water for 12 hours and passed through the chopper. Mix with almond or sesame puree sauce or yoghurt sauce. For dried fruits, always look for good quality without preservatives or bleach; otherwise, gastrointestinal problems may occur.

Bircher muesli with condensed milk*
If you do not have almond or sesame puree or fresh yoghurt at hand, you can make the muesli with condensed milk according to the original recipe. Disadvantage: Condensed milk often contains sugar.

Fruit and fresh grain dishes

Fresh grain cereal mash with banana
2 tsp cereal meal
½ banana
1 tsp honey
lemon as desired

Soak chopped cereal for 12 hours, then mix. Crush the banana with a fork and add it. Flavour with honey and lemon juice. Serve at once.

Fresh whole grain with berries
1 level tbs freshly ground wholemeal grains (wheat, rye, oats)
1 tbs water
1 tbs honey
lemon juice as desired
100 g berries (any kind)

Soak wholemeal grains for approx. 6 hours. Crush berries with a wooden spoon or mix with honey and lemon juice and mix into the grains.

Fresh whole grain with orange juice
1 level tbs freshly ground wholemeal grains (wheat, rye, oats)
1 tbs water
1 tbs honey
1 dl orange juice
1 tbs ground nuts

Soak wholemeal grains for approx. 6 hours. Mix in honey, orange juice and nuts. The fresh, unblended whole grain can also be soaked and mixed in.

Sprouted cereal grains
These are very high in the vitamin E and B group, and generally have a strengthening effect.
1st day, evening: wash the grains in a colander under running water and place them in a bowl.
Cover with water and keep at room temperature, close to the oven.
2nd day, morning: rinse the grains and spread to dry on a flat plate. Keep at room temperature, close to the oven.
Evening: put the grains back in the bowl and cover with water. Keep at room temperature, close to the oven.
3rd day, morning: rinse the grains and spread to dry on the plate.
The same evening put the grains back in the bowl and cover with water. Keep at room temperature, close to the oven.
On the 4th day, the grains should have developed sprouts 1–2 cm long and are ready to eat.

The preparation of sprouted cereal grains is easier to accomplish in the practical sprouting devices that are available in various sizes.
Sprouted cereal grains are suitable to prepare muesli but also as an addition to salads or raw vegetables.

Chilled soups

Chilled soup
1 tsp honey
1 tsp agar-agar powder
1–1.5 dl water
2 peaches
or berries
or stone fruit
or pomes

Cook honey with agar-agar until the powder has completely dissolved. Cut the peaches finely and pour some lemon juice over them to keep them from turning brown. Leave the berries whole, chop stone fruit or pomes.
Pour the sauce over the fresh fruit and allow it to cool.

Milk types

Almond milk
This food provides vegetable protein and oil and is rich in valuable unsaturated plant oils. Stimulates mucous production and is soothing.

2 tsp almond puree ½ tsp honey
2 dl water

Whisk almond puree and honey and water.

Almond milk of fresh almonds
Very easy to digest.

1½ tsp almonds, peeled (no bitter almonds)
½ tsp honey
2 dl water

Mix almonds, honey and water in the mixer. Strain if necessary.,

Pine nut milk

Very rich in easily digestible vegetable oils and protein that protects the metabolism.

1½ tsp pine nuts, washed
1 tsp honey
1 ½ dl water

Prepare as for almond milk.

Sesame milk
Rich in high-quality fatty acids.

2 dl water (cold or warm)
1 level tbs sesame puree
1 tsp lemon juice
1 tsp honey

Whisk sesame puree, honey and the water. Add the lemon juice last.

Sesame cream
Like sesame milk, but with less water added. Replaces cream in cooked dishes and desserts.

Sesame frappé (milkshake)
Like sesame milk or sesame cream, with addition of fruit juice, apple juice, fruit concentrates.

Soy milk
1 cup soy beans
7 cups water
1 tbs fruit sugar water
Wash and dry soy beans and grind them in an almond mill. Soak for 2 hours then boil for 20 minutes in the water used for soaking, stirring constantly. Strain. Add water until the viscosity of cow's milk is reached. Add fructose and let cool. Soy milk is sold in tetra packs in health food stores.

Raw vegetables and salads

There are three conditions to be respected when preparing raw vegetables and salads:

1. Freshness and quality
For any other diet and for full everyday nutrition, use only sun-ripened, organically grown vegetables and salads. They are not only ideal for health, but also taste best. Today the offer from businesses run in accordance with organic guidelines is very extensive, and organically grown vegetables are available in many supermarkets. Vegetables and salads from your own garden are, of course, ideal. Herbs and tomatoes can be grown even on a balcony. Choose young, tender leafy lettuces and root vegetables, unblanched, and remove any wilted leaves or rotting stalks. For a healing regime it is important to use only entirely fresh plants of the best quality.

Prepare raw vegetables just before eating them, and mix them with the dressing immediately. Unless used immediately, chopped vegetables and salads rapidly lose their vitamin content.

2. Cleanliness
Vegetables grown organically without the use of artificial fertilizers contain no worm eggs. Nevertheless, all fresh plants must be cleaned thoroughly and carefully. Observe that water soluble substances such as Vitamin C, vitamins of the B group and minerals are leached out in water.

3. Harmonious composition
Every salad dish should contain all three types of vegetables: root, fruit and leaf. Green leafy lettuce in particular is always part of a healing regime. In the dressings, variety is desirable for the different ingredients of the raw food diet. A beautifully assembled salad in pleasing colours is

agreeable to the eye and the palate, and stimulates the appetite. Small garnishes of herbs, radishes, young carrots or olives make the raw vegetable dish even more colourful and festive. In everyday use the three kinds of vegetables per meal should not be exceeded. Too much variety may impair digestion.

Cleaning leafy vegetables
For head lettuce, endives, romaine lettuce, iceberg lettuce and similar green leaf lettuces, cabbage and red cabbage, etc. separate the leaves and clean them individually and carefully under running water. Rinse several times and dry thoroughly in a salad spinner.
Small-leaved salads such as lamb's lettuce and cut lettuce, spinach, dandelion, cress, rocket, radicchio and Brussel's sprouts should be rinsed repeatedly in small portions, and any hard stalks should be removed. Halve chicory/endive, remove outer leaves and rinse well.

Cleaning root vegetables
Celery root (celeriac), carrots, horseradish, radish, beetroot, kohlrabi, black salsify: clean with a brush under running water, peel and immediately grate or slice into the finished sauce. Mix well to preserve the vegetables' fresh colour.

Cleaning vegetable fruits
Wash tomatoes and cut them into wedges or slices. Peel cucumbers and cut them small or grate them. Organically grown young cucumbers do not need to be peeled.
Use only young, tender unpeeled courgettes for salads, wash them thoroughly, then slice or julienne them.
Green and yellow sweet peppers are milder than the red variety.
Wash, halve, remove seeds and dice. Unfortunately, almost all non-organic sweet peppers now come from hydroponic production.

Separate cauliflower and broccoli into florets, and clean thoroughly under running water.
Wash stalk celery, peel when necessary, and cut away hard parts.
Halve leeks and fennel, prepare and wash under the spray tap.

Salad dressings

Use the various dressings as prescribed by a doctor.

Oil dressing (mild)
1 tbs oil (rapeseed, sunflower or olive oil from first cold pressing, thistle oil, walnut oil, add 50 % flaxseed oil)
1 tsp lemon juice or organic fruit vinegar optional garlic, pressed
1 tsp fresh herbs (or knife tip dried herbs)

Mix all the ingredients and whisk the dressing until creamy. The dressing also is even tastier with a splash of soy sauce or Kelpamare.
This classic salad dressing is suitable for all green salads (head lettuce, romaine lettuce, cress, etc.) and fruit salads (tomatoes, cucumbers etc.).

Quark dressing*
1 tbs lean quark
3 tsp butter milk
½ tsp fresh lemon juice, finely chopped herbs

Whisk all ingredients thoroughly.
This dressing goes particularly well with root vegetables (carrots, celery root (celeriac), radishes, etc.).

Yoghurt dressing*
For low fat diet.
2–3 tsp yoghurt
a few drops of lemon juice, onion, grated (optional)
a little garlic, pressed (optional)
1 tsp fresh herbs (or knife tip dried herbs)

Whisk all ingredients thoroughly.
A refreshing dressing with cress or spinach, with fruit salads (tomatoes, cucumbers) and with root vegetables (kohlrabi, horseradish, radishes).

Cream dressing*
2 tsp sour cream
1 tsp lean quark
1 tsp lemon juice, very little pepper
1 tsp fresh herbs (or knife tip dried herbs)

Whisk all ingredients thoroughly.
This dressing goes well with almost all root and fruit salads. For a change, you may replace lemon juice with orange juice to give the raw food a new flavour. With celery root (celeriac), beetroot and chicory/endive salad, you may add a little freshly ground horseradish to this dressing for a very stimulating taste.

Almond puree or sesame puree dressing (mild)
1 tbs almond or sesame puree
3 tsp water
1 tsp lemon juice
a little garlic, pressed (optional)
1 tsp fresh herbs
(or knife tip dried herbs)

Slowly stir sesame or almond puree with water until smooth, then add the other ingredients.
This tasty dressing is very suitable for root vegetables.

Classic mayonnaise recipe*
For 4 persons:
1 egg yolk
1 tbs lemon juice
2 dl oil
onion, herbs, a little Kelpamare

Mix the egg yolk well with several drops of lemon juice. Add the oil drop by drop while whisking evenly. If the mayonnaise becomes too thick, dilute with lemon juice. Season to taste.

For 1 portion:
1 tbs mayonnaise
1 tsp lemon juice
1 tsp fresh (or 1 knife-tip of dried herbs)
Mix all ingredients well.

Mayonnaise with wholegrain soy flour instead of egg (mild)
For 6–8 portions.
2 tsp soy wholegrain flour
6 tsp water
2 dl oil

Mix soy wholegrain flour and water until smooth. Slowly add oil while constantly stirring with the whisk.
The mayonnaise can be kept in the refrigerator for a few days.

For 1 portion you need:
1 tbs mayonnaise
1 tsp lemon juice
a touch of mustard (optional)
1 tsp fresh herbs (or knife tip dried herbs)

Mix all ingredients well. Mayonnaise is a popular dressing for salads composed of field and root vegetables.

Raw vegetables, mixed
Chicory/endive with diced tomato and oil dressing or mayonnaise
sweet pepper and fennel – oil dressing
fennel, chicory/endive, diced tomato and mayonnaise*
fennel and carrots – cream dressing or mayonnaise*
cauliflower and carrots – cream dressing or mayonnaise*
tomatoes and peppers – oil dressing

Tomatoes, raw, stuffed
with cucumbers – oil dressing
with celery root (celeriac) – cream dressing*
with cauliflower – cream dressing*

Sauerkraut salad
Sauerkraut is a particularly wholesome raw vegetable, especially in winter. It is more easily digestible raw than cooked, and has a gallbladder-purging and disinfecting effect. Use low salt organic sauerkraut if possible. An addition of finely-cut raw sauerkraut can considerably improve the taste and digestive qualities of steamed sauerkraut. For a salad, the sauerkraut is loosely separated and chopped, mixed with a few caraway seeds (or ground caraway), 3–4 chopped juniper berries, chopped onion, a julienned apple or a diced small fresh pineapple. Choose oil dressing as a dressing. This salad goes particularly well with corn salad and a raw root vegetable.

Mixed – pureed raw vegetables
If the doctor prescribes a 'pureed diet', certain raw vegetables may be mixed with the dressing in the blender. This is the transition from juice to normal raw vegetable food. The pureed vegetables must be eaten immediately after being spooned in and blended.

Examples:
1 tomato 70 g
1 handful spinach 30 g
1 small carrot 70 g
one knife-tip marjoram
with oil dressing

1 tomato 70 g
1 handful head lettuce 20 g
1 small piece of celery root (celeriac) 20 g
with cream dressing
(with lovage)

beetroots 30 g
zucchini 40 g
head lettuce 20 g
with cream dressing (with dill)*

celery root (celeriac) 40 g
carrots 40 g
spinach 20 g
almond puree dressing
(with rosemary)

Suggestions for dressings to go with the salads and raw vegetables

head lettuce	uncut	oil dressing	chives, onion
cut lettuce	uncut	oil dressing	chives, onion
chicoy/endive	cut in strips of 1 cm	oil dressing	onion, parsley
lamb's lettuce	uncut	oil dressing	onion, parsley
cress	uncut	yoghurt dressing	chives
spinach	cut strips of ½ cm	yoghurt dressing	peppermint
cabbage lettuces: white cabbage, sauerkraut, Brussels sprouts, savoy cabbage	slice, cut into thin pieces	oil dressing or mayonnaise	lovage, savory, thyme, caraway
tomatoes	slice or dice	oil dressing or yoghurt dressing	basil, thyme, oregano
cucumbers	slice	oil dressing	dill
aniseed	finely cut with knife	cream dressing or oil dressing	dill, chives, parsley
sweet peppers	cut into fine strips	oil dressing or mayonnaise	chives
radish	slice or grate	quark dressing	chives, parsley
radishes	slice or cut finely	yoghurt dressing	chives, parsley
stalk celery	cut finely	oil dressing or almond puree dressing	chives, thyme
courgettes	grate coarsely or slice	oil dressing or almond puree dressing	dill, borage, basil
carrots	grate finely	yoghurt or orange dressing	chives, lovage
celery root (celeriac)	grate finely	cream sauce	ginger
beetroot	grate finely	cream sauce	horseradish
cauliflower, broccoli	cut off florets, grate stems	garlic dressing	chives
endive/chicory	cut in strips of 1 cm	cream sauce	tarragon, parsley
Jerusalem artichoke	grate	mayonnaise	marjoram, thyme
kohlrabi	slice or grate	yoghurt dressing or cream dressing	thyme, lovage
red cabbage	slice or cut finely	almond puree dressing	some grated apple, caraway, lovage

Chives, parsley and onions may be added in moderation to any raw vegetable, according to taste.

Cooked food

Such food is only used after the first healing phase, i.e. after the first two dietary levels of raw food. Every meal must still begin with raw food. In particular in the summer months, when convenient, fresh juice and raw food days should also be used intermittently. The following cooked food should not make up more than one-third of the volume of the raw food eaten previously.

Recipes that contain animal protein and fat are marked with an asterisk (*). These may be used if one wants to prevent neurodegenerative diseases. However, someone who is suffering from a neurodegenerative disease should not use these recipes, since animal fats and proteins have to be avoided. Cream may be replaced by soy cream or almond puree.

Garlic, a very important ingredient, is used mainly with raw food, since it loses much of its health-giving effect when heated, and the cooked recipes taste better with onions.

Every meal should begin with fruit and nuts. Breakfast and dinner should be small and as frugal as possible, as at the first and second raw food dietary level. One should drink only while eating the fruit, and repeatedly between the meals. Drinking with the fruit will send the fruit directly to the duodenum, which will promote digestion and development of the proper intestinal flora.

The recipes for cooked meals have been designed in accordance with the very valuable experience gained at the original Bircher-Benner hospital. They appeal to the taste and are readily digestible. They correspond to a whole food diet as created by Dr. Maximilian Bircher-Benner, who also coined the term 'whole food'.

The cooking times are indicated without the use of a pressure cooker or a steamer, and can be reduced to approx. one-third or one-fourth if such a device is used. This is highly recommended.

Recipes for cooked food

Soups
All recipes are for 1 person.

The following soup and vegetable recipes require a large amount of vegetable broth. In a small household, it is inconvenient to make fresh vegetable broth every day. Instead, you may use ordinary water and salt-free vegetable bouillon cubes or pastes.
In case of wheat allergy, the wholegrain flour in the recipes should be replaced by rice, millet or oat flour.

Vegetable broth
As the only exception, this recipe is for 4 persons.

1 tbs organic nut spread or olive oil
1 onion
2 carrots
1 small stalk of celery (150 g) cabbage, Swiss chard leaves
1 leek stalk
3–4 l water
½ bay leaf
1 pinch rock salt
lovage, basil or other herbs, dried or preferably fresh

Halve the onion, keeping the brown peel, and brown the cut area in the hot fat. Chop the vegetables, add and cook for at least 15 minutes covered at low heat. Add water and cook for 2 hours at low heat. Season to taste.

Vegetable bouillon
3 dl vegetable broth
a pinch of rock salt (optional)

10 g nut spread or olive oil
parsley, chives, freshly chopped herbs

Prepare the vegetable broth according to the above recipe and add to nut spread, vegetable fat and herbs. Add more rock salt to taste.

Semolina dumplings*
10 g butter
1½ tsp fine semolina
½–1 egg
1 pinch rock salt
marjoram, nutmeg
6 dl vegetable broth

Cream the butter until foamy. Mix the semolina and egg thoroughly with the butter. Add salt and spices and let the mix stand for 30 minutes. Use a teaspoon to shape the dumplings. Place them in the boiling vegetable bouillon and steep for 15 to 20 minutes.

Rice soup, clear
½ tbs olive oil or organic nut spread
a little chopped onion
1 small carrot
a little celery root (celeriac) and leek
1 tbs rice
1 pinch rock salt
6 dl vegetable broth
chives

Sauté onion with finely cut vegetables and rice. Add hot vegetable broth and cook for 15–20 minutes. Prepare with finely cut chives and vegetable fat.

Rice soup, thickened
½ tbs organic nut spread
a little celery root (celeriac)
1 small carrot
a little leek
1 tbs rice
½ tbs wholegrain flour
6 dl vegetable broth or water lovage,
parsley, basil,
marjoram

a little soya sauce (optional)
½ tbs cream* or sesame cream (see recipe page 102)
chives

Sauté the chopped vegetables in the fat. Sprinkle with wholegrain flour, add the vegetable broth and cook for 30 minutes. Season with soy sauce and herbs. Place cream and finely cut chives in the soup bowl and serve the soup over them.

Oat cream soup
½ tbs organic nut spread or olive oil
2 tsp fine or coarse oat flakes
6 dl vegetable broth or a little celery root (celeriac)
½ tbs cream* or sesame cream (recipe see page 102)
optional: miso, chives, nutmeg or caraway

Briefly sauté oat flakes with or without vegetable fat. Add vegetable broth and celery root (celeriac). Slightly cook oat flakes for 10 minutes (coarse oats must be cooked for at least 20 minutes). Season to taste. Place cream or sesame cream and chives in the soup bowl and add the pureed soup.

Oat groat soup
½ tbs organic nut spread or olive oil
2 tsp oat groats
chopped onion
8 dl water or vegetable broth
a little diced celery root (celeriac)
1 pinch stone salt or little miso
chives, parsley, marjoram or borage

Sauté onion and groats with or without vegetable fat. Add vegetable broth and celery root (celeriac) and cook for 45–60 minutes. Season to taste with stone salt or miso. Place herbs in the soup bowl and add the soup.

Tomato soup
½ tbs organic nut spread or olive oil
a little onion, celery root (celeriac) and leek

1 small carrot
1 garlic clove
1 tomato
1 tbs wholegrain flour
6 dl vegetable broth
1 pinch rock salt
tomato puree (optional)
1 pinch fruit sugar
rosemary, oregano
5 g organic nut spread
½ tbs cream* or sesame cream (recipe see page 102)
chives

Sauté diced vegetables with or without vegetable fat, then add the tomato. Sprinkle with wholegrain flour and add vegetable broth. Cook for ½ hour then strain. Add spices and optional tomato puree. Place olive oil or nut spread and cream (optional) in the soup bowl, and add the finished soup. Sprinkle with finally cut chives. If desired, add 1 tablespoon rice to the soup or sprinkle with fat-free toasted bread cubes (croutons).

Summer tomato soup
4 ripe tomatoes
1 pinch fruit sugar
1 pinch rock salt
½ tbs cream* or sesame cream (recipe see page 102)

Dice the tomatoes, cook briefly, season and strain. Add the cream or sesame cream and serve the soup lukewarm or cold.

Vegetable soups (carrots, spinach, broccoli, cauliflower)
½ tbs organic nut spread or olive oil
a little chopped onion
1½ tsp wholegrain flour
1 pinch rock salt
6 dl vegetable broth
1 tbs cream* or sesame cream (recipe see page 102)
Vegetables: 1 diced carrot or 1 small cup of spinach pureed or finely chopped, broccoli or cauliflower finely chopped (cook some of the flowers separately and set them aside).

Sauté onion and carrots or broccoli with or without olive oil. Sprinkle with wholegrain flour and sauté them briefly. Pour in vegetable broth and cook for 20–40 minutes. For the spinach soup, add the spinach last and remove from heat. Pour the soup over the cream or sesame cream in the soup bowl. For the broccoli and cauliflower soup, add the flowers previously set aside.
Seasoning the vegetable soups:
For carrot soup, use celery leaves or lovage, rosemary or marjoram, 1 teaspoon caraway.
For spinach soup, use peppermint leaves, parsley, chives, pinch of nutmeg.
For broccoli or cauliflower soup, use a little basil, parsley, chives, tarragon.

Chervil soup*
½ tbs organic nut spread or olive oil
a little onion
1 medium-sized potato, chopped in cubes
½ tbs wholegrain flour
5 dl vegetable broth
1 pinch rock salt
1 tbs chervil, chopped
½ tbs cream* or sesame cream (recipe see page 102)

Sauté the onion slightly with or without vegetable fat. Add potato, sprinkle with wholegrain flour and add vegetable broth and a pinch of salt. Cook for ½ hour and strain. Put chervil and cream or sesame cream in the soup bowl and add the soup.

Potato soup
½ leek, cut into thin strips
½ carrot, sliced
½ tbs wholegrain flour 5 dl vegetable broth
1 medium-sized potato, diced
1 pinch rock salt or some miso,
basil, marjoram

½ tbs cream* or sesame cream (recipe see page 102)

Sauté the leek and carrot in a little vegetable broth. Sprinkle with wholegrain flour and add the vegetable broth. Add potato and cook until soft. Season to taste. Place basil, marjoram and optional cream or sesame cream in the soup bowl and add the finished soup.

Minestrone
½ tbs organic nut spread or olive oil
2 tbs leek
a little onion, finely chopped
a few celery leaves
½ plate mangold leaves
7 dl water or vegetable broth
1 tbs lovage or thyme
½ garlic clove, pressed
basil, parsley, chives
1 pinch rock salt
15 g pasta or rice
5 g nut spread or 1 tsp olive oil

Mince onion, leek, celery leaves and mangold leaves and sauté them slowly. Add vegetable broth, season and cook for 30 minutes. Add pasta or rice and cook another 15–20 minutes. To enhance flavour, add nut spread or olive oil.

Vegetables

Spinach, chopped
¼ l vegetable broth
200 g spinach (remove thick stems)
¼ garlic clove, pressed
1 pinch rock salt
peppermint leaves, sage
1 cup raw spinach
little optional fresh butter* or organic nut spread

Briefly cook spinach in the vegetable broth and drain, then cut, chop or blend. Return spinach to the pan and heat. Add garlic, salt and herbs. Chop or blend the raw spinach and add to the cooked spinach (with a little butter, olive oil or nut spread) before serving.

Spinach, whole leaves (and stems)
300 g spinach (remove thick stems, briefly boil the coarser winter spinach if required)
1 tbs pine nuts
1 tbs raisins (optional)
1 pinch rock salt
peppermint leaves, sage, parsley optional
melted butter* or organic nut spread or olive oil

Sauté spinach uncovered over low heat with a little water.
Add pine nuts, spices and optional raisins and briefly continue cooking. Add liquid butter, olive oil or nut spread to taste.

Lettuce
1 romaine lettuce
1 l water
a little chopped onion
½ tbs organic nut spread or olive oil
1 dl vegetable broth
1 pinch rock salt
2 tsp cream* or sesame cream (recipe see page 102)

Halve the romaine lettuce, boil until softish then drain. Reassemble the lettuce and place in an oven-proof baking dish. Lightly sauté the onion with nut spread or olive oil and place it over the lettuce. Add vegetable broth and a pinch of rock salt and cook in the oven for 30–40 minutes. Add the cream or sesame cream 5 minutes. before serving.

Sautéed chicory (endive)
2 heads chicory/endive
½ tbs organic nut spread or olive oil
3 tsp vegetable broth
1 pinch rock salt marjoram, thyme
Halve the chicory/endive and layer the leaves in the pan. Add heated nut spread or olive oil and vegetable broth to the

chicory/endive, season and cook covered over low heat for 30 minutes. Spread melted nut spread or little olive oil on the prepared vegetables.

Celery stalks
3–4 stalks celery
½ onion, chopped
a little apple, finely chopped
1 dl vegetable broth
1 tsp almond puree
1 pinch rock salt or a little soya
celery greens

Cut the celery stalk into pieces 8 cm long and place in a pan. Briefly sauté the onion and apple without fat and spread over the celery. Add vegetable broth and almond puree and cook over low heat for ½ to ¾ hour. Season.

Baked fennel with cream cheese sauce*
1 large or 2 small fennel plants
1 pinch rock salt
pepper
several drops of lemon juice
1 cream cheese

Quarter the fennel and steam it until semi-soft. Pull apart the individual layers of the fennel bulb and place them in an oven-proof mould. Drizzle with lemon juice then add salt and pepper. Stir the cream cheese with 2 tablespoons of fennel stock and spread over the vegetables. Bake in hot oven.

Vegetable curry
1 tbs olive oil
1 spring onion
200 g vegetables (e.g. leeks, carrots, courgettes, asparagus)
½ tsp wholegrain flour
1 knife tip (to taste) curry powder
½ tsp vegetable broth
½ orange
1 tsp sultanas
1 pinch whole sugar
1 pinch rock salt, pepper

Cut the spring onion into fine rings and cook in slightly heated oil. Sprinkle on flour and curry powder and add the vegetable broth. Add the cut vegetables and cook covered for approx. 15 minutes. Set aside two or three wedges of the orange, squeeze the rest and place the sultanas in the juice. When the vegetables are soft, add the sultanas and orange juice, heat the mixture and season with sugar, salt and pepper. Serve and spread the orange wedges on top.

Cooked carrots
3–4 carrots
1 dl vegetable broth
1 tsp almond puree
1 pinch each fruit sugar and rock salt
marjoram, thyme, rosemary, parsley

Cut the carrots in strips or rounds and cook in the vegetable broth for 30–45 minutes. Stir in the almond puree (optional). Season and sprinkle the chopped parsley.

Peas and carrots
½ tbs organic nut spread or olive oil
100 g fresh peas, shelled
1 dl vegetable broth
marjoram, thyme, lovage
parsley, chives

150 g sliced carrots, prepared according to the above recipe for cooked carrots
Briefly sauté peas in the nut spread or olive oil, add vegetable broth and cook until soft. Season. Mix carrots and peas or serve them alternately on the platter.

Cooked sugar peas (snow peas) (mange tout)
200 g snow peas
1 dl vegetable broth
1 pinch rock salt
1 pinch whole sugar
a little parsley or lovage
organic nut spread or olive oil

Cook sugar peas and herbs covered in the vegetable broth for ½ to ¾ hour. Season and add olive oil or nut spread when serving.

Green beans with tomatoes
½ tbs organic nut spread or olive oil
½ onion
250 g beans
a little garlic
savoury, parsley
1 – 2 tomatoes
1 pinch rock salt
caraway, marjoram, lovage

Sauté the chopped onions in organic nut spread or olive oil. Sauté the beans, finely diced tomatoes and herbs for approx. 1 hour. Add water if necessary. Season to taste.

Steamed celery root (celeriac)
½ tbs organic nut spread or olive oil
½ onion
½ celery root (celeriac)
1 dl vegetable broth
1 pinch rock salt
a little lemon juice, marjoram
1 tsp almond puree
very thin slices of apple, nuts

Sauté the chopped onions in organic nut spread or olive oil. Add the julienned celery root (celeriac) and vegetable broth and cook until soft, ½ to ¾ hour. Season. To refine, add almond puree and, if desired, apple slices. Sprinkle with chopped nuts.

Stewed tomatoes
4 – 5 tomatoes
½ tbs organic nut spread or olive oil
½ onion
fruit sugar
1 pinch rock salt
touch of garlic
rosemary, marjoram, basil
1 tbs corn starch (optional)
parsley or chives or dill

Slightly brown onion and fruit sugar in nut fat or olive oil. Douse the tomatoes with boiling water then peel them, cut them into pieces, add them to the onions and cook the mixture until slightly thickened. Add garlic and spices and finish cooking (add corn starch to thicken). Sprinkle chopped parsley or other herbs abundantly on the prepared tomatoes.

Steamed tomatoes
2 – 3 tomatoes
1 pinch rock salt
10 g organic nut spread or olive oil
¼ onion, chopped
herbes de Provence (basil, rosemary, thyme, sage)
parsley

Sauté the onion without fat. Put the halved tomatoes on a greased tray or ovenproof dish. Add dabs of nut spread or rub olive oil on each tomato half, and spread the sautéed onion and herbs on it. Cook briefly in the oven.
Some tomatoes may be minced or very finely chopped, blended with cream*, parboiled briefly and spread over the prepared tomato.

Tomatoes à la Provençale
2 tomatoes
1 pinch rock salt
1 tbs chopped parsley
1 tbs breadcrumbs

Halve tomatoes, sprinkle with rock salt, and place on a tray. Mix breadcrumbs and parsley and spread on the tomatoes with a spoon. Bake in the oven for 15 minutes.

Courgettes with tomatoes
½ tbs organic nut spread or olive oil
½ onion, chopped
300 g courgette
50 g tomato
1 pinch rock salt
garlic, rosemary, marjoram, thyme, basil

parsley, chive, dill
maize flour (optional)
1 tsp almond puree

Simmer onion in vegetable fat. Dice the courgettes; peel and dice the tomatoes. Add the vegetables to the onions and cook until soft. Season to taste. If there is too much liquid, add stirred maize flour and 1 teaspoon almond puree before serving.

Sweet peppers (green, yellow, red)
These are very suitable as an addition to other dishes.
150–200 g sweet peppers
½ tbs organic nut spread or olive oil
½ onion, chopped
1 pinch rock salt
garlic, rosemary, marjoram, thyme
basil, parsley

Cut the sweet peppers in strips and sauté them in nut spread or olive oil with the onion, herbs and spices in a covered pan for at least ½ hour.

Ratatouille
50 g sweet peppers
100 g courgette
50 g aubergine
1 tomato
½ onion, chopped
a little garlic
1 tbs organic nut spread or olive oil
1 pinch rock salt
rosemary, marjoram, thyme, basil
parsley

Chop the sweet peppers, courgettes, aubergines and tomato (peeled). Sauté onion and garlic in nut spread or olive oil, add vegetables and cook covered for 1 hour. Season. If there is too much sauce, leave it to thicken while covered.

Aubergines
Wash the aubergines, peel (optional)
1 tbs organic nut spread or olive oil
400–500 g aubergines
a little vegetable broth (optional) rock salt
1–2 tomatoes

Steam the aubergines, cut into cubes, and sauté in nut spread or olive oil until soft. Salt as allowed. Garnish with a few tomato halves or with stewed tomatoes.

Artichokes
1 artichoke
¾ l water
1 tbs lemon juice
1 pinch rock salt

Cut off the stalks close to the artichokes themselves. Remove the bottommost hard leaves and remove the tips. Halve and cut out the heart; wash under running water and rub the cut surface with lemon juice. Bring water to the boil, add lemon juice and rock salt, and cook the artichoke until soft for approx. ¾ h.
Drain and serve the artichoke on a warm platter covered with a serviette.
Serve with vinaigrette (see recipe page 121).

Asparagus
½ asparagus bunch
1 l water
1 pinch rock salt
grated cheese*
nut spread or olive oil

Wash the asparagus and peel the stalks thoroughly. Green asparagus can be left almost whole. Cook the asparagus in boiling water for 20–30 minutes until soft (quicker with green asparagus), remove with a slotted skimming spoon and serve on a platter covered with a serviette. Sprinkle cheese* and pour liquid nut spread or olive oil over the dish.
As a variation, serve with vinaigrette sauce (see recipe page 121).

Cauliflower or broccoli
Only from organic production.
1 small cauliflower or
broccoli (250 g)
1 tsp organic nut spread or olive oil
1 garlic clove
1 dl vegetable broth
1 pinch stone salt, pepper
pine nuts or almond slices

Cut off the leaves and stalk below the flower. Peel the stalk and cut into larger pieces; divide the flower into florets. Lightly brown the chopped garlic clove in nut spread or olive oil, add the cauliflower or broccoli and sauté briefly. Cover with vegetable broth and cook for approx. 5 minutes. Season with salt and pepper. Briefly roast pine nuts or sliced almond in a pan without fat and spread on the vegetables.

Cabbage or white cabbage, steamed
(Do not eat cooked cabbage if you are suffering from flatulence. Cabbage does not cause flatulence when raw. All cabbages must be chewed well; raw cabbage juice is always permitted and does not cause flatulence.)
½ tbs organic nut spread or olive oil
½ onion, chopped
250 g young cabbage
1 dl vegetable broth
nutmeg, caraway, 1 pinch stone salt
basil or lovage

Sauté onions in nut spread or olive oil. Cut cabbage in strips 2 cm wide, add to the onions and cook until the vegetables begin to soften. Add vegetable broth and cook over low heat for 30 minutes until soft. Season to taste.
Green, mature cabbage must be blanched before cooking.

Red cabbage
(Avoid if suffering from meteorism.)
½ tbs organic nut spread or olive oil
250 g red cabbage
½ tsp lemon juice
½ apple
½ tbs rice
1 dl vegetable broth
½ dl grape juice or apple juice
1 apple
a little butter*
1 pinch rock salt

Steam the finely grated red cabbage in vegetable fat. Add lemon juice, apple cut into fine slices and rice. Continue steaming. Add vegetable broth and grape juice or apple juice and steam until soft, covered over low heat for 1–1½ hours. Peel the second apple, cut into wedges. Add butter and braise the apple wedges on a tin baking sheet in the oven. Garnish the prepared red cabbage with the apple wedges.

Salads of cooked vegetables

Carrots, celery root (celeriac), beetroot, beans, cauliflower, broccoli, courgettes, mangold leaves and Swiss chard are particularly suitable for these salads.
The vegetables are cooked in vegetable broth or water until soft, drained and cut small (diced, sliced, florets, strips). Serve with salad dressing or with vinaigrette or mayonnaise. Enhance with onions and chopped herbs.

Potato salad
200 g potatoes
½ dl vegetable broth
1 tbs mayonnaise or mayonnaise with wholegrain soy flour instead of egg (see recipe page 104)*
½ tbs chopped onions
borage, chives, parsley
lemon balm, marjoram, thyme, dill

Cook the potatoes until soft in the pressure cooker, peel while hot and slice. Pour the heated vegetable broth on them and let stand for a short time, then mix in the mayonnaise*. Season with onions and herbs. Mayonnaise can be replaced with oil, lemon juice and cream, well mixed and added to the potatoes.

Potato salad with cucumbers
1 large potato
¼ cucumber
2 tsp yoghurt sauce (see recipe page 103)*
½ garlic clove
dill or borage, chives
parsley, onion

Prepare the potato as described above. Coarsely grate the peeled cucumber and add to the potato. Mix with yoghurt sauce and season with onions and herbs.
Rub the salad bowl with the garlic clove before serving.

Salade niçoise*
1 boiled potato
1 small tomato radishes
several cucumber slices
1 hardboiled egg*
1 tbs olive oil
½ tbs lemon juice
1 pinch rock salt
parsley, chives or dill
lemon balm, borage
a few leaves of head lettuce

Slice the potato, tomato, radish and egg and, together with the cucumber slices, top with a salad dressing of oil, lemon juice, rock salt and herbs. Just before serving, cut the leaves of head lettuce into broad strips and mix with the salad or prepare the salad on the head lettuce leaves.

Vegetable aspics
½ dl vegetable broth 2 g agar-agar
a few drops of lemon juice
a little rock salt
fresh slices of cucumber, cubes of tomato
broccoli flowers, cooked
peas, cooked
beans, cooked and finely chopped

Agar-agar is plant-based gelatine powder that is used for vegetable and fruit aspics, sauces and puddings, etc. instead of animal gelatine.
Add agar-agar powder to the lukewarm vegetable broth and heat slowly until the gelling agent is thoroughly dissolved. Season with lemon juice and a little rock salt. Pour a little aspic into the rinsed moulds and let it harden. Garnish with vegetable slices, add more aspic, let it harden and repeat until the moulds are filled.
Turn over the cooled aspics and serve on a bed of salad leaves.

Potato dishes

Potatoes in their skins
3–4 small potatoes, water
Brush and wash potatoes. Fill pan with steamer insert or wire screen with water up to the insert, add potatoes, cover and cook for 30–40 minutes (8–10 minutes in the pressure cooker).

Baked potatoes (jacket potatoes)
3–4 small potatoes
1 tbs olive oil
butter*, nut spread or olive oil

Brush and wash the potatoes. Score the peel on the top 3–4 times, brush with oil and bake the potatoes on a greased sheet at medium heat for 30–40 minutes. Put a dab of butter* or nut spread on each of the cooked potatoes or brush with little olive oil.

Caraway potatoes
2–3 medium-sized, longish narrow potatoes
1 tsp caraway
1 pinch rock salt
1 tbs olive oil

Wash and clean the potatoes and cut them in half crosswise. Mix caraway with rock salt and sprinkle on the cut side of the potatoes. Place the potatoes with the cut side down on a greased tray, brush with olive oil and bake at medium heat for ¾ hour.

Bouillon potatoes
250 g potatoes
1–2 dl vegetable broth
1 pinch rock salt
lovage, thyme
10 g butter*, organic nut spread or olive oil

Wash potatoes, peel, halve or cut into pieces and cook until soft in the vegetable broth with the salt and spices. Spread butter or nut spread on the prepared potatoes or brush with olive oil.

Potatoes with tomatoes
200 g potatoes
½ small onion
1 dl vegetable broth
1 small tomato
1 pinch rock salt
½ tbs cream* or sesame cream (recipe see page 102)
marjoram, rosemary or thyme

Briefly sauté the chopped onion and peeled, sliced potatoes without fat, then cook them in the vegetable broth until softish. Cut the peeled tomato into wedges, add and finish cooking. Season to taste. Add the cream or sesame cream before serving.

Mashed potatoes
4 potatoes
water
dried tomatoes
butter* or organic nut spread or olive oil

Wash, peel, quarter and steam the potatoes until soft. Rice the potatoes onto a warm plate. Add liquid butter, nut spread or olive oil and garnish with minced dried tomatoes.

Roast potatoes
2 small potatoes
water for steaming
1 pinch rock salt
1 dl vegetable broth
1–2 tsp cream* or sesame cream (see recipe page 102) or nut spread
nutmeg, thyme
parsley

Peel and halve potatoes and steam them until softish. Put them on an oven-proof dish with the cut side down. Cover with vegetable broth. Season and roast in the oven until the liquid has thickened. Add cream or nut spread and continue roasting until the potatoes are lightly browned. Serve with the cut facing up and sprinkle with chopped parsley.

Lyonnaise potatoes
1 tbs organic nut spread
½ tbs olive oil
3 small potatoes
1 small onion

Organic margarine and oil. Peel potatoes and cut into slices. Cook in liquid fat until softish. Add sliced onion and finish cooking.

Ayurveda potatoes
(An attractive, aromatic dish that yields 3–4 helpings)
5 large potatoes
½ soy drink
1 package of soy cream (substitute for crème fraîche)
1 bunch each of fresh dill, fresh chives and fresh parsley
juice of ½ lemon
1–2 tsp turmeric
½ tsp curry
soy sauce

Cut the cleaned potatoes into thick slices and cook them for approx. 5 minutes. In the meantime, slowly heat the soy drink in a pan, mixed with the soy cream (do not boil). Stir in turmeric and curry to taste and season with soy sauce. Put the potato slices in the sauce and simmer for approx. 10 minutes. Sprinkle the fresh, finely chopped herbs on the potatoes and serve at once.

Cereal dishes

Japanese rice
80 g wholegrain rice
1½–2 dl vegetable bouillon
1 pinch rock salt
10 g organic nut spread or olive oil
1 small peeled onion studded with clove and bay leaf

Put the rice and studded onion in the bouillon and boil for 40 minutes. Leave to cool and remove the onion. Reheat the rice in the oven and top with heated nut spread or olive oil before serving.

Risotto
80 g wholegrain rice
½ tbs organic nut spread or olive oil
1 tbs chopped onion
2 dl vegetable broth or water
1 pinch rock salt
dried mushrooms
fresh herbs to taste
rosemary
10 g fresh butter* or nut spread
10 g Parmesan cheese* (optional)

Sauté onion in the margarine, add rice and sauté until rice is translucent. Add the vegetable broth or hot water and cook until al dente (30–40 minutes). Add the finely chopped, dried mushrooms and herbs and cook briefly. Before serving, mix in butter, nut spread or olive oil and grated Parmesan cheese with a fork.

Saffron rice
Prepare like risotto. Dissolve a knife tip of saffron powder in a little bouillon and add to rice.

Riz creole with vegetables
½ tbs organic nut spread or olive oil
80 g wholegrain rice
2 tsp diced vegetables
(leeks, celery root (celeriac), carrots)
2 dl vegetable broth
1 pinch rock salt
freshly chopped herbs to taste

Briefly sauté rice and vegetables, add hot vegetable broth and herbs, and cook for 30–45 minutes.

Tomato rice
80 g wholegrain rice
½ tbs organic nut spread or olive oil
1 tbs chopped onion
a little garlic, pressed
approx. 1 dl vegetable broth
1 pinch rock salt
rosemary, marjoram, nutmeg
basil (optional)
whole cane sugar
10 g organic nut spread or olive oil

Sauté onion and garlic in nut spread or olive oil, add rice and sauté until the rice is translucent. Add peeled, diced tomato. Add vegetable broth and spices and cook for 30–45 minutes. Add nut spread or olive oil before serving.

Rice with courgettes
½ tbs organic nut spread
80 g wholegrain rice
1 tbs onion, chopped 150 g tender courgettes
1 pinch rock salt
1½ dl vegetable broth or water
freshly chopped dill
10 g organic nut spread or olive oil

Dice the courgettes. Prepare dish as for tomato rice (see above).

Rice with spinach
80 g wholegrain rice
½ tbs organic nut spread or olive oil 100 g spinach

onion, chopped
2 dl vegetable broth or water
1 pinch rock salt
nutmeg and peppermint
10 g nut spread

Cut spinach coarsely. Prepare dish as for tomato rice (see above).

Rice with peas (Risi bisi)
80 g wholegrain rice
150 g garden peas, shelled
½ tbs organic nut spread or olive oil
onion, chopped
1 pinch each fruit sugar and rock salt
½ dl vegetable broth
1½–2 dl water
10 g nut spread
parsley

Sauté onion with fruit sugar and a pinch of salt in the margarine. Add the peas and cook briefly, then add vegetable broth and cook the peas until soft. Prepare risotto (according to the above recipe) in a separate pan. Add the peas to the cooked risotto. Before serving, top the prepared rice with nut spread or olive oil and chopped parsley.

Indian rice
80 g wholegrain rice
2 dl vegetable broth
1 pinch rock salt
1 small banana
1 small apple
1 tbs raisins
1 tsp sunflower seeds
1 tsp sesame seeds
saffron, curry, fresh ginger root

Cook rice with vegetable broth and 1 pinch of rock salt until not quite soft (approx. 30–40 minutes). Mix the sliced banana, the peeled and sliced apple, and the raisins into the rice and continue boiling for 5–10 minutes. Season with saffron, curry and ginger root to taste. Sprinkle with sunflower seeds and lightly dry-roasted sesame seeds (without fat).

Polenta
½ tbs olive oil
50 g maize semolina, medium fine
3 dl water
nutmeg
1 pinch rock salt
½ tbs organic nut spread or olive oil

Oil pan. Boil water and stir in the maize. Boil for 5 minutes over low heat, stirring frequently. Season and continue boiling for 45–60 minutes over low heat. Add nut spread or olive oil before serving. You may also add onion slices sautéed without fat.

Millet risotto with vegetables
40 g millet
1 tbs onion, chopped
2 tsp finely chopped vegetable cubes (leek, celery root (celeriac), carrots or carrots and peas)
½ dl vegetable broth
a little rock salt
rosemary
1 tbs grated cheese* (optional)
10 g fresh butter* or nut spread

Sauté onion, diced vegetable and hot-rinsed millet until glazed. Add hot vegetable broth, season and boil for 20 minutes. When serving, add grated cheese* (optional) and a little butter, nut spread flakes or olive oil.

Coarse-ground grain mash
2 tsp coarse-ground grain (wheat, oats, rye)
3 tsp water
1 pinch rock salt

Soak the coarse-ground grain for 12 hours. Then boil in water for 10 minutes or cook for ½ h. in a bain-marie. Salt to taste.

Pasta, spaghetti, macaroni, etc.
For a curative diet, egg pasta should not be used. Today there are high quality wholegrain pastas, soy pastas and spelt pastas in addition to the well-known Italian pasta products made from wheat. There are also many ready-prepared sauces, though these usually contain too much fat (oil, butter, cheese, cream).
The most easily digested pasta products are cooked al dente with a classic or simple tomato sauce (see recipes in the chapter 'Sauces').

Spätzle or Knöpfli (without egg)
60 g wholegrain flour
20 g soy flour
1 dl 1:1 diluted milk
1 l water
1 pinch rock salt
1 tbs organic nut spread or olive oil
onion, julienned
chives and parsley

Mix wholegrain and soy flour thoroughly with diluted milk and knead the mixture until the dough forms bubbles. Leave to stand for at least 1 hour.
Boil water with rock salt. Press the dough in portions through a coarse screen into the boiling water or place it on a small wooden cutting board. Cut fine strips with a knife and place them in the boiling water. Let the Knöpfli or Spätzle simmer until they rise to the surface. Take them out with a skimmer and place them on a hot platter. As desired, garnish with julienned onion sautéed in nut spread (or without fat), chives and parsley.

Spinach or tomato Knöpfli*
70 g wholegrain flour (⅓ soy flour)
1 egg*
1 dl 1:1 diluted milk
1 handful of chopped, raw spinach
1 tsp tomato puree
1 dl water
1 pinch rock salt
chives and parsley

Make a smooth batter from the wholemeal and soy flour, egg and water, and leave to stand for 1 hour. Prepare and cook Knöpfli or Spätzle according to the recipe above. Add spinach or tomato puree. Season with chives and parsley.

Oat flake roasts
½ tbs of health store nut spread
1 tbs chopped onion
2 tsp of chopped leek, celery, spinach
50 g oat flakes
½ dl vegetable broth
nut spread or olive oil
peppermint or sage

Steam onions and vegetables in nut spread or olive oil, add oat flakes and vegetable broth and cook to a thick mash. Season. Spread approx. 1 cm high on a board and leave to cool. Cut into rectangles. Heat nut spread or olive oil and toast both sides to a golden yellow.

Spinach omelette*
50 g wholegrain flour
1 egg*
100 g milk water
Rock salt
25 g raw, chopped spinach
10 g health store nut spread

Process all ingredients into a smooth dough and leave to stand. Bake omelettes in the heated nut spread.

Sauces

Sauces are a challenge for those on a healing diet, since almost all sauce recipes contain a large amount of fat (butter, oil, cream), cheese and eggs. The combination of hot fat and flour (classic béchamel sauce) should always be avoided. We have put together a few permissible sauces here, whose recipes differ from the classical ones. All of them taste really great.

Béchamel sauce without egg (recipe 1)
For 4 persons:
2–3 tsp wheat flour
1 l milk* or water
1 bay leaf
1 tbs vegetable broth
1 grated onion
1 pinch each rock salt, nutmeg and freshly ground white pepper
chopped parsley

Briefly cook the flour without fat until it is aromatic (it must not turn dark), then let cool slightly. Add the milk or water, bay leaf, vegetable broth and onion while stirring constantly. Bring to the boil. Season to taste. After approx. 5 minutes, remove the bay leaf and serve the sauce sprinkled with parsley.

This basic sauce can be used to make many versions. For example:
Horseradish sauce: When completed, add 10 grammes finely grated horseradish and cook the sauce for another 5 minutes.
Caper sauce: Season the finished sauce with whole or chopped capers and lemon juice.
Olive sauce: Briefly cook the sauce with 4–5 tablespoons tomato puree and 2 tablespoons chopped olives. Season with a knife point of cayenne pepper (optional).
Herb sauce: Add a large quantity of finely chopped herbs such as parsley, lovage, chervil, basil, estragon, oregano, etc. into the finished sauce.
Mushroom sauce: Mix 3–4 tablespoons of very finely chopped raw mushrooms into the finished sauce and season with lemon juice.

Béchamel sauce (recipe 2)
For 4 persons:
2 tsp wheat flour
½ l soy milk
1 bay leaf
1 onion, finely grated
2 tsp red miso
1 pinch each of pepper, paprika and chopped parsley

Briefly brown the flour without fat until it gives off a toasted aroma. Leave to cool briefly then add the soy milk while stirring constantly. Add the bay leaf and onion and boil for about 5 minutes.
Stir in the miso, remove the bay leaf and season the sauce with pepper and paprika. Sprinkle with chopped parsley.
Miso is a fermented soybean paste that is excellent for seasoning. It tastes like soy sauce but does not contain table salt.

Tomato sauce, classic
½ tbs organic nut spread or olive oil
1 tbs onion
½ garlic clove, pressed
2 tsp carrot, celery root (celeriac), leek
2 small tomatoes
1 pinch rock salt
1 pinch whole sugar
1 tsp tomato puree
1½ dl vegetable broth or water
bay leaf, rosemary, thyme

Sauté the chopped onion, pressed garlic and coarsely cut vegetables in nut spread or olive oil. Add the diced tomatoes and the tomato puree, then add vegetable broth (or water). Season and simmer for ½ hour. Strain if desired.

Tomato sauce, simple
3 tomatoes
1 pinch each rock salt and raw cane sugar
chives, basil
1 tbs olive oil

Dice tomatoes, sauté until soft, season and drain. Add olive oil to taste.

Classic mayonnaise recipe*
For 4 persons:
1 egg yolk*
1 tbs lemon juice
2 dl oil
1 pinch rock salt, onion, herbs

Beat the egg yolk thoroughly with several drops of lemon juice. Add the oil drop by drop while stirring evenly with the whisk. If the mayonnaise is too thick, dilute with lemon juice. Season to taste.

Remoulade sauce, classic*
For 4 persons:
Prepare mayonnaise according to above recipe
1 hardboiled egg*, chopped
1 tbs cornichons, chopped
1 tsp parsley, chopped
tomato, diced

Mix the various ingredients with the finished mayonnaise. Garnish with diced tomato.

Mayonnaise without animal protein and fat
See recipe page 104.

Remoulade sauce without animal-based protein
For 4 persons:
Prepare mayonnaise without animal-based protein and fat (see recipe page 104) and mix with 1 tablespoon chopped cornichons, capers and chopped parsley. Garnish with diced tomato.

Vinaigrette*
For 4 persons:
1 tbs olive oil
2 tsp ground nut oil
2 ½ tsp lemon juice
2 tsp water or vegetable broth
½ onion, chopped
1 egg*, hardboiled and chopped
1–2 cornichons, cut or finely chopped
parsley or chives
1 tbs small tomato, diced
1 pinch rock salt

Whisk oil, lemon juice and vegetable broth until smooth, then add the other ingredients, while mixing thoroughly. The egg is optional.

Sandwiches

Sandwiches are popular as appetizers and summer meals, and to take along on hikes and journeys.
Spreads and ingredients can be used in any number of ways, and various wholegrain types of bread are available, some pre-sliced.
Remember that many loaves are made just to look 'wholegrain' by means of artificial colouring and added grains.
Do use real wholemeal bread or pumpernickel.
The recipes are for 4 persons.

Basic spreads
For the strict diet, simply spread organic nut spread on the bread rolls and fill with raw food.

Guacamole (avocado mousse)
2 ripe avocados
juice of ½ lemon
½ small chopped onion
2 garlic cloves, pressed
rock salt and white pepper (optional)

Mash the flesh removed from the avocados together with the lemon juice in a blender. Add the onion and garlic and season with rock salt and white pepper. If desired, stir in 1 tablespoon soy cream (instead of crème fraiche).

Sweet avocado cream
1 ripe avocado
4 tsp fresh orange juice
1 tbs honey
1 knife tip ginger powder

Mash the removed pulp of the avocado by squeezing it out or blending it and mix in the other ingredients.
Serve at once.

Tofu spread with nuts
250 g tofu, pureed
2 finely chopped spring onions

50 g nuts (hazelnuts, walnuts, almonds, cashew nuts)
rock salt and white pepper (optional)

Lightly roast the nuts in the oven or a dry pan, let cool. Grind the roasted nuts and mix with the pureed tofu and onion. Season with rock salt and pepper.

Quark spread with herbs*
100 g quark
10 g organic nut spread
miso or some rock salt
caraway, chives or herbs (dill, borage, lovage, basil, oregano, peppermint etc.)

Stir quark and nut spread to a frothy consistency, season and add individual herbs (or a mix) for variety.

Garnishes
Spreads can be garnished in the following ways:
with raw carrots or celery root (celeriac), with tomatoes, fresh cucumbers, radish, cress, onion rings, nuts, parsley, chives etc.

Recipes Index

Almond milk	101
Almond milk of fresh almonds	101
Almond puree or sesame puree dressing	104
Artichokes	113
Asparagus	113
Aubergines	113
Avocado mousse (Guacamole)	121
Ayurveda potatoes	116
Baked potatoes (jacket potatoes)	115
Béchamel sauce (recipe 2)	120
Béchamel sauce without egg (recipe 1)	120
Bircher muesli	99
Bircher muesli with almond or sesame puree (vegan)	99
Bircher muesli with berries or stone fruit	100
Bircher muesli with condensed milk	100
Bircher muesli with cream	100
Bircher muesli with dried fruits	100
Bircher muesli with various fruits	100
Bircher muesli with yoghurt, sour milk or buttermilk	99
Bouillon potatoes	116
Cabbage or white cabbage, steamed	114
Caper sauce	120
Caraway potatoes	115
Cauliflower or broccoli	114
Celery stalks	111
Cereal dishes	117
Chervil soup	109
Chilled soup	101
Classic mayonnaise recipe	104, 120
Coarse-ground grain mash	118
Cooked carrots	111
Cooked sugar peas (snow peas) (mange tout)	111
Courgettes with tomatoes	112
Cream dressing	104
Fennel, baked with cream cheese sauce	111
Flaxseed gruel	99
Fresh grain cereal mash with banana	100
Fresh whole grain with berries	100
Fresh whole grain with orange juice	101
Fruit and fresh grain dishes	100
Fruit juices	98
Garnishes	122
Green beans with tomatoes	112
Gruel to accompany juices	99
Guacamole (avocado mousse)	121
Herb sauce	120
Horseradish sauce	120
Indian rice	118
Japanese rice	117
Juices	98
Lettuce	110
Lyonnaise potatoes	116
Macaroni	119
Mashed potatoes	116
Mayonnaise without animal protein and fat	121
Mayonnaise with wholegrain soy flour instead of egg (mild)	104

123

Milk types	101
Millet risotto with vegetables	118
Minestrone	110
Mixed – pureed raw vegetables	105
Mushroom sauce	120
Oat cream soup	108
Oat flake roasts	119
Oat groat soup	108
Oil dressing (mild)	103
Olive sauce	120
Pasta	119
Peas and carrots	111
Pine nut milk	102
Polenta	118
Potato dishes	115
Potatoes in their skins	115
Potatoes with tomatoes	116
Potato juice	99
Potato salad	114
Potato salad with cucumbers	115
Potato soup	109
Quark dressing	103
Quark spread with herbs	122
Ratatouille	113
Raw vegetables and salads	102
Raw vegetables, mixed	104
Red cabbage	114
Remoulade sauce, classic	121
Remoulade sauce without animal-based protein	121
Rice or barley gruel	99
Rice soup, clear	108
Rice soup, thickened	108
Rice with courgettes	117
Rice with peas (Risi bisi)	118
Rice with spinach	117
Risi bisi (rice with peas)	118
Risotto	117
Riz creole with vegetables	117
Roast potatoes	116
Saffron rice	117
Salad dressings	103
Salade niçoise	115
Salads and raw vegetables	102
Salads of cooked vegetables	114
Sandwiches	121
Sauces	119
Sauerkraut salad	105
Sautéed chicory (endive)	110
Semolina dumplings	108
Sesame cream	102
Sesame frappé (milkshake)	102
Sesame milk	102
Soups	107
Soy milk	102
Spaghetti	119
Spätzle or Knöpfli (without egg)	119
Spinach, chopped	110
Spinach omelette	119
Spinach, whole leaves (and stems)	110
Sprouted cereal grains	101
Steamed celery root (celeriac)	112
Steamed tomatoes	112
Stewed tomatoes	112
Summer tomato soup	109
Sweet avocado cream	121
Sweet peppers (green, yellow, red)	113
Tofu spread with nuts	121
Tomatoes à la Provençale	112
Tomatoes, raw, stuffed	104
Tomato rice	117
Tomato sauce, classic	120
Tomato sauce, simple	120
Tomato soup	108
Vegetable aspics	115
Vegetable bouillon	107
Vegetable broth	107
Vegetable curry	111
Vegetable juices	98
Vegetable soups (carrots, spinach, broccoli, cauliflower)	109
Vinaigrette	121
Yoghurt dressing	103

Notes

1. Endepols, H. et al., 'Effort based decision making in the rat: A (18F) fluodeoxiglucose micro positron emitting tomography study', *J Neurosci* 20 (29) 2010, pp 7908–14.
2. Di Paolo et al., 'Chronic exposure to aluminium and melatonin through the diet: neurobehavioral effects in a transgenetic mouse model of Alzheimer disease', *Food Chem toxicol*. 2014 July, 69 pp 320–29.
3. Huppelsberg, J. et al., *Kurzlehrbuch der Physiologie*, 4th edition, Thieme-Verlag, p 223.
4. Ransohoff, R.M. et al., 'The myeloid cells of the central nervous system parenchyma', *Nature* 468, no 7312, 2010, pp 253–62. PMID 21068834.
5. Fagerholm, U., 'The highly permeable blood-brain barrier: an evaluation of current opinions about brain uptake capacity', *Drug discovery today* 12, 2007, pp 1076–82. PMID 18061888 (review).
6. Chiu, W.L. et al., 'Linear correlation of the fraction of oral dose absorbed of 64 drugs between humans and rats', *Pharm Res* 15, 1998, pp 1792–95. PMID 9834005.
7. Goodwin, U.T. et al., 'In silico predictions of blood-brain barrier penetration: considerations to "keep in mind"', *J pharmacol Exp ther* 315, 2005, pp 477–83. PMID 15919767 (review).
8. Mato, M. et al., 'Evidence for the possible function of the fluorescent granular perithelial cells in brain as scavengers of high-molecular marker ED-2', *Experientia* 40, 1984, pp 399–402. PMID 6325229.
9. Balabanov, R. et al., 'CNS vascular pericytes express macrophage-like function, cell-surface integrin alpha M, a macrophage marker ED-2', *Microvasc Res* 52, 1996, pp 127–42. PMID 8901442.
10. Hickey, W.F. et al., 'Perivascular microglial cells of the CNS are bone-marrow derived and present antigens in vivo', *Science* 239, 1988, pp 290–92. PMID 3276004.
11. Fabry, Z. et al., 'Differential activation of Th1 and Th2 CD4+ cells by murine brain microvessel endothelial cells and smooth muscle pericytes', *J Immunol* 151, 1993, pp 38–47. PMID 8100844.
12. Täuble, H., 'Carriers and specificity in membranes. E. Carrier facilitates transport. Kinks as carriers in membranes', *Neurosci Res Program Bull* 9, 1971, pp 361–372. PMID 5164654.
13. Träuble, H., 'Phasenumwandlungen in Lipiden. Mögliche Schaltprozesse in biologischen Membranen', *Naturwissenschaften* 58, 1971, pp 277–284. PMID 4935358 (review).
14. Vastowsky, O.,:'Chemie der Naturstoffe-Lipoproteine und Membranen' (http://www.chemie.uni erlangen.de/0c/vostrowsky/naturstoff/03 Membranen. pdf), Universität Erlangen, 2005, p 42.
15. Timai, I. et al., 'Structure internalization relationship for adsorptive mediated endocytosis of basic peptides at the blood-brain barrier', *J Pharmacol Exp Ther* 280, 1997, pp 10–15. ONUD 8996222.
16. Weiss, N. et al., 'The blood-brain barrier in brain homeostasis and neurological diseases', *Biochem. Biophys. Acta* 1788, 2009, pp 842–57 (review).
17. Banks, W.A. et al., 'Cytokines and the blood-brain-barrier', Siegel, A. et al., 'The neuro-immunological basis of behavior and mental disorders', *Springer*, New York, 2009, pp 3–17.
18. Hill, H.U., 'Umweltschadstoffe und neurodegenerative Erkrankungen des Gehirns', *Demenzkrankheiten*, Shaker-Verlag Aachen 2010, pp 62–63.
19. Comford, E.M. et al., 'Comparison of lipid-mediated blood-brain-barrier permeability in neonates and adults', *Am J Physiol-Cell Physiol* 243, 1982, pp 161C–68C. PMID 7114247.
20. Elmas, I. et al., 'Effects of profound hypothermia on the blood-brain barrier in brain homeostasis and neurological diseases', *Forensic Science International* 119, 2001, pp 212–16. PMID 11376985.

21 Phillips, S.C. et al., 'Weakening of the blood-brain barrier by alcohol-related stresses in the rat', *J Neurol Sci* 54, 1982, pp 271–78. PMID 7201507.
22 Sing, A.K. et al., 'Effects of chronic alcohol drinking on the blood-brain barrier and ensuing neuronal toxicity in alcohol-preferring rats subjected to intraperitoneal LPS injection', *J Neurol Sci* 54, 1982, pp 271–78. PMID 7201507.
23 Haorah, J. et al., 'Alcool-induced blood-brain-barrier dysfunction is mediated via inositol 1,4,5-triphosphate receptor (IP3R)-gated intracellular calcium release', *J Neurochem* 100, 2007, pp 324–336. PMID 1724115.
24 Haorah, J. et al., 'Ethanol-induced activation of myosin light chain kinase leads to dysfunction of tight junctions and blood-brain barrier compromise. Alcoholism', *Clinical and Experimental Research* 29, 2005, pp 999–1009. PMID 15976526.
25 Haorah, J. et al., 'Alcohol induced oxydative stress in brain endothelial cells causes blood-brain barrier dysfunction', *J of Leukocye Biology* 78, 2005, pp 1223–32. PMID 16204625.
26 Peters, R. et al., 'Smoking, dementia and cognitive decline in the elderly, a systematic review', *BMC Geriatr* 8, 2008, p 36. PMID 19105840 (review).
27 Lockman, P.R. et al., 'Brain uptake kinetics of nicotine and cotinine after chronic nicotine exposure', *J Pharmacol Exp Ther* 314, 2005, pp 636–642. PMID 15845856.
28 Chen, Y.H. et al., 'Enhanced Escherichia coli invasion of human brain microvascular endothelial cells is associated with alternations in cytoskeleton induced by nicotine', *Cell Microbiol* 4, 2002, pp 503–14. PMID 12174085.
29 D'Andrea, D.A. et al., 'Microwave effects on the nervous system', *Bioelectromagnetics* 6, 2003, pp 107–174. PMID 14628310 (review).
30 Patel, T.H. et al., 'Blood-brain barrier dysfunction associated with increased expression of tissue and urokinase plasminogen activators following peripheral thermal injury', *Neurosci Lett* 444, 2008, pp 222–26. PMID 18719505.
31 Salford, L.G. et al., 'Nerve cell damage in mammalian brain after exposure to microwaves from GSM mobile phones', *Environ Health perspect* 111, 2003, pp 881–883. PMID 12782486.
32 Nittby, H. et al., 'Radiofrequency and extremely low-frequency electromagnetic field effects on the blood-brain barrier', *Electromagn Biol Med* 27, 2008, pp 215–229. PMID 18821198.
33 Eberhardt, J.L. et al., 'Blood-brain barrier permeability and nerve cell damage in rat brain 14 and 28 days after exposure to microwaves from GSM mobile phones', *Electromagn Biol Med* 27, 2008, pp 215–229. PMID 18821198.
34 Salford, L.G. et al., 'Permeability of the blood-brain barrier induced by 914 MHz electromagnetic radiation, continuous wave and modulated at 8, 16, 50 and 200 Hz, *Microsc Res Tech* 2727, 1994, pp 245–542. PMID 8012056.
35 Meyl, K., 'Elektromagnetische Umweltverträglichkeit', *Umdruck zum Informationstechnischen Seminar*, Indel GmbH Verlagsabteilung Villingen-Schwemmingen, 2002, 3rd edition, pp 81–83.
36 Patel, J.R. et al., 'Moderators of Oligodendrocyte differentiation during remyelinisation', doi:10.1016/j.febslet.2011.04.037.
37 Shen, S. et al., 'Age dependent epigenetic control of differentiation inhibitors is critical for remyelinisation efficiency', *Nature Neurosciensce* 11(9), pp 1024–34.
38 Hanafy, K.H. et al., 'Regulation of Remyelinisation in multiple sclerosis', *FEBS-letters* 585(23) pp 3821–3828.
39 Franklin, R.J.M. et al., 'Remyelinisation in the CNS: from biology to therapy', *Nature Reviews Neuroscience* 9(11) pp 839–55.
40 Herold, G., *Lehrbuch der Inneren Medizin* 2010, p 836.
41 Dittmann, S., 'Risiko des Impfens und das noch grössere Risiko, nicht geimpft zu sein', *Bundesgesundheitsblatt-Gesundheitsforschung-Gesundheitsschutz* 2002, no. 45, pp 316–322.
42 Burns, T.M., 'Guillain-Barré Syndrome', *Semin Neurol.* 2008: Apr 28(2), p 154. PMID 18351518.
43 Merlini, G. et al., 'Molecular mechanisms of amyloidosis', *N Engl J Med* no 349, 2003, pp 583–96.
44 Van Vijck, R. et al., Utrecht University: 'An introduction to Human Biophoton Emission', *Forsch Komplementärmed Klass Naturheilkd.* 2005, 12 pp 77–83.
45 Gurwitsch, A.G., *Das Problem der Zellteilung*, Springer-Verlag, Berlin, 1926; *Die mitogenetische Zellstrahlung*, Springer-Verlag Berlin, 1932, Ferner; 'Arch R. mikr. Anat. Und Entwicklungsmech', vols 51, 52, 100, 101 and 104.

46. Bischof, M., *Biophotonen, das Licht in unseren Zellen,* ISBN 3-86150 095 7.
47. Popp, F.A., *Biologie des Lichtes, Grundlagen der ultraschwachen Zellstrahlung,* Verlag Paul Parey, ISBN: 3-489-61734-7.
48. Rubik, B., 'Natural light from organisms: life at the edge of sciences', in Fischer, H. 'Photons as transmitters for intra- and extracellular biological and biochemical communication: the construction of a hypothesis', *Electromagnetic Bio-Information,* Popp, F.A. ed., Urban und Schwarzenberg, Munich, 1989, p 70.
49. Bircher-Benner, M.O., *Grundzüge der Ernährungstherapie auf Grund der Energie-Spannung der Nahrung,* Verlag Otto Salle, Berlin, 1905 and 1906.
50. Bircher-Benner, M.O., 'Der zweite Hauptsatz der Energetik und die Ernährung', *Zschr der Wendepunkt,* Wendepunkt-Verlag, Zürich, 1936 and 'Vom Wesen und der Organisation der Nahrungs-energie und über die Anwendung des zweiten Hauptsatzes der Energielehre auf den Nährwert und die Nahrungswirkung', *Kleine Hippokrates-Bücherei,* vol 8, Hippokrates-Verlag Stuttgart and Leipzig, 1936.
51. Popp, F.A., *Unsere Lebensmittel in neuer Sicht,* ISBN 3-596-11459-4.
52. Prigogine, I. et al., *Dialog mit der Natur,* Piper-Verlag München, ISBN 3-492-11181-5.
53. Kasnaceev, C.P. in Jezowska-Trzebiatoveska, B. et al., 'Photon emission from biological systems', proceedings of the first international symposium, Wroclav Pland Jan 1986.
54. Harman, D., 'Aging: a theory based on free radical and radication chemistry', *J of Gerontology* 11, 1956, pp 298–300. PMID 13332224.
55. Harman, D., 'The free radical theory of aging', *Antioxid Redox Signal* 5, 2003, pp 557–561. PMID 14580310.
56. Bockman, K.B. et al., 'Mitochondrial aging: open questions', *Ann N.Y. Acad Sci* 854, 1998, pp 118–127. PMID 9928425.
57. Sohr, Ch., 'Oxydativer Stress bei diabetischer Neuropathie', Medizinische Fakultät, Deutsches Diabetes-Zentrum DDZ 2007 (online).
58. Berg, D. et al., 'Parkinson's disease', in Lajita, A. et al., *Handbook of Neurochemistry and molecular Neurology,* 3rd edition: *Degenerative Diseases of the Nervous System,* Springer-Verlag, Berlin, Heidelberg, 2007, p 9ff.
59. Kilburn, K.H., 'Neurobehavioral and pulmonary impairment in 105 adults with indoor exposure to molds compared to 100 exposed to chemicals', *Toxicol. Ind. Health* 25 (9–10) pp 681–92.
60. Hill, H.U., 'Umweltschadstoffe und Neurodegenerative Erkrankungen des Gehirns', *Demenzkrankheiten,* Shakefr-Verlag Aachen, 2010, p 5.
61. Schäfer, S.G. et al., *Metalle, Lehrbuch der Toxikologie,* Wiss. Verlagsgesellschaft mbH Stuttgart, 2nd edition 2003, p 273ff.
62. Birkmeyer, J.D.D. et al., 'Quecksilberdepots im Organismus korrelieren mit der Anzahl der Amalgamfüllungen'. Deutsche Zeitschr für Biologische Zahnmedizin 6, pp 57–61.
63. Mutter, J. et al., *Amalgam-Risiko für die Menschheit. Quecksilbervergiftungen richtig ausleiten. Fit fürs Leben-Verlag,* 2nd edition, Natura Viva Verlags-GmbH, Weil der Stadt, 2006.
64. Drasch, G. et al., 'Mercury burden of human fetal and infant tissues', *Eur. J. Paediat.* 1994(8), pp 607–10.
65. Olivieri, G. et al., 'The effects of β-estradiol on SHSY6Y neuroblastome cells during heavy metal induced oxidative stress, neurotoxicity and β-Amyloid secretion', *Neuroci* 113 pp 849–55.
66. Griem, P. et al., 'Metal-induced autoimmunity', *Curr Opin Immunol* 7 pp 831–39.
67. Grandjean, P. et al., 'Cognitive deficit in seven-year-old children with prenatal exposure to methylmercury', *Neurotox Toxicol* 19, pp 417–28, 1997.
68. Dott et al., *Lehrbuch der Umweltmedizin,* Wiss. Verlagsgesellschaft Stuttgart 2002, p 170ff.
69. Curth, A., 'Der Einfluss von Quecksilber auf die Entstehung der Alzheime-Erkrankung: eine systematische Review', medical dissertation, Universitätsklinik Freiburg i.B., 2008, http://www.freidoc.uni-freiburg.de/volltexte/6091.
70. Mutter, J. et al., 'Quecksilber und Alzheimer Krankheit', *Fortschr Neurol Psychiatr* 75, pp 528–38.
71. Greenpeace: dpa Meldung 2000.
72. Schäfer, S.G. et al., *Lehrbuch der Toxikologie,* Wiss. Verlagsgesellschaft mbH. Stuttgart, 2nd edition 2003, p 763ff.
73. Hill, H.U., 'Umweltschadstoffe und Neurodegenerative Erkrankungen des Gehirns', *Demenz-*

erkrankungen, Shaker-Verlag, Aachen, 2nd edition.

74 Haga, S. et al., 'Neuronal degeneration and glia-cell responses following trimethylin intoxication in the rat', *Acta Neuropathol* 103 (6), pp 575–82.

75 Binz, P., 'Zehn Fallberichte (Kasuistiken) von Patienten mit Chemikalienbelastung (Organophosphatpestizide, Reinigungsmittel mit Chlorgehalt) aus der neurologischen Praxis', in Hill, H. U., 'Umweltschadstoffe und Neurodegenerative Erkrankungen des Gehirns', *Demenzkrankheiten*, Shaker-Verlag Aachen, 2010, p 17.

76 Axelson, O. et al., 'A case-referent study on neuro-psychiatric disorders among workers exposed to solvents', *Scand J Work Environ Health* 2 pp 14–20.

77 Husmann, K., 'Symptoms of car painters with long-term exposure to organic solvents', *Scand J Work Environ Health* 6, pp 19–26.

78 Schwartz, E., 'Proportionate mortality ration analysis of automobile mechanics and gasoline service station workers in New Hampshire', *Am J Ind Med* 12, pp 91–99.

79 Ashford, N.A. et al., 'Chemical exposures: low levels and high stakes', *Toxicol Ind Health* 3, pp 1–7.

80 Merz, T. et al., 'Merkblatt zur Bewertung von VOC-Gemischen', *Umwelt-Medizin-Gesellschaft* 18/4, 2005, pp 291–93.

81 UBA, 'Richtwerte für Innenraumluft', in Eikmann et al, *Gefährdung: Toxikologische Basisdaten und ihre Bewertung,* Erich Schmidt-Verlag, Berlin, 2002.

82 Binz, P., 'Zehn Fallberichte (Kasuistiken) von Patienten mit Chemikalienbelastungen (Organophosphat-Pestizide, Reinigungsmittel mit Chlorgehalt) aus der neurologischen Praxis', in Hill, H. U., 'Umweltschadstoffe und Neurodegenerative Erkrankungen des Gehirns', *Demenzkrankheiten*, Shaker-Verlag, Aachen, 2010, pp 23–24.

83 Hörr, B., 'Positronen-Emissions-Tomographie (PET)-Befunde von 2 Patienten mit Organophosphat-Pestizid Belastung', in Hill, H. U., 'Umweltschadstoffe und neurodegenerative Erkrankungen des Gehirns', *Demenzkrankheiten*, Shaker-Verlag, Aachen, 2010 pp 23–24.

84 Sayal, et al., 'Prenatal alcohol exposure and gender differences in children's mental health problems: longitudinal population-based study, *Pediatrics* 119(2) 2002, pp 426–34.

85 Alkohol, 'Das fetale Alkoholsyndrom' (http://www.fasworld.eu/home.html).

86 *Süddeutsche Zeitung,* 'Jedes Jahr 10 000 Babies mit Alkoholschaden', 9 September 2008, p 12.

87 Crellin, R. et al., 'Folates and psychiatric disorders, Clinic potential', *Drugs* 45, 1993 (45) pp 623–36.

88 Herrmann, W., *Mitochondriale Medizin Teil 12*: 'Homocystein und Neurodegeneration', online article in www.ganzimmun.de, 31 May 2010 (online seminar archive).

89 Durk, M.R. et al., '1α-25-Dihydroxyvitamin D3 reduces cerebral amyloid-β-accumulation and improves cognition in mouse models of Alzheimer's disease', *J Neuropsy* 2014 May 21, 34(21) pp 7091–101.

90 Groves, N.J. et al., 'Vitamin D as a neurosteroid affecting the developing and adult brain', *Annu Rev Nutr* 2014, 34 pp 117–41.

91 Kfoszynnska, M. et al., 'The role of vitamin D in multiple sclerosis', *Postepy Hit Med Dosw* (online) 2015 April 8, 69 pp 440–6.

92 Schwarz, S. et al., 'Diet and multiple sclerosis', *Nervenarzt* 2005 Feb 76 (2) pp 131–42.

93 Flachenecker, Z. et al, 'Epidemiologie', in Schmidt and Hofmann (Hrsg.), *Multiple Sklerose,* Urban und Fischer, München 2002, ISBN 3-437-22080-2, pp 4–11.

94 Evangelou, G.C. et al., 'Pathological study of spinal cord atrophy in multiple sclerosis suggests limited rule of local lesions', in *Brain: a journal of neurology*, vol 128, pt 1.1.2005, pp 29–34.

95 Kutzelnigg, C.F. et al., *Cortical demyelinization and diffuse white matter injury in multiple sclerosis.*

96 In *Brain, a journal of neurology*, vol 128, pt 11, Nov 2005, pp 1705–12.

97 Bernhard, L., 'Neuronale Degeneration bei spinaler multipler Sklerose', medical school dissertation, Charité-Universitätsmedizin Berlin, 2010.

98 Lundmark, F. et al., 'Variation in interleukin 7 receptor alpha chain (IR7R) influences risk of multiple sclerosis', *Nature genetics* 39, no 9, Sept 2007, pp 1108–1113.

99 Morrosu, M.G. et al., 'Susceptibility to multiple sclerosis: the role of interleukin genes', *The Lancet neurology*, vol 6, no 10 Oct 2007, pp 846–7.

100. Sawcer, S., 'The complex genetics of multiple sclerosis: pitfalls and prospects'. *Brain*, vol 131, pt 12, Dec 2008, pp 3118–31.

101. Gregory, A. P. et al., 'TNF-receptor 1 genetic risk mirrors outcome of anti-TNF therapy in multiple sclerosis', *Nature*. vol 488, no 7412, Aug 2012, pp 508–11.

102. Patsopoulos, N. A. et al., 'Fine-mapping the genetic association of the major histocompatibility complex in multiple sclerosis: HLA and non-HLA effects', *PLOS Genetics* vol 9, no 11, Nov 2013, p e1003926.

103. Bashinskaya, V. et al., 'A review of genome-wide association studies for multiple sclerosis: classical and hypothesis-driven approaches', *Hum Genet* 2015 Nov, 134(11–12), pp 1143–62.

104. Bhatia, R. et al., 'Epidemiology and genetic aspects of multiple sclerosis in India', *Ann Indian Acad Acad Neurol* 2015 Sept 18 suppl1 pp 6–10.

105. Dyment, D. A., 'Multiple sclerosis in stepsiblings: recurrence risk and ascertainment', *J neurology, neurosurgery and psychiatry*, vol 77, no 2, Feb 2006, pp 258–9.

106. Banwell, B. et al., 'Clinical features and viral serologies in children with multiple sclerosis: a multinational observational study', *Lancet neurology*, vol 6, no 9, Sept 2007, pp 773–81.

107. Alotaibi, S. et al., 'Epstein-Barr Virus in pedatric multiple sclerosis', *JAMA* vol 291, no 15, April 2004, pp 1875–79.

108. Mori, M., 'Association between Multiple Sclerosis or Neuromyelitis Optica and Epstein-Barr Virus', *Brain Nerve* 2015 Jul, 67(7) pp 881–90.

109. Pfuhl, C. et al., 'Association of serum Epstein-Barr nuclear antigen-1 antibodies and intrathecal immunoglobulin synthesis in early multiple sclerosis', *J Neuroimmunol* 2015 Aug 15, 285 pp 156–60.

110. Galiero, A. et al., 'Detection of Mycobacterium avium subsp. paratuberculosis in cheese from small ruminants in Tuscany', *Int J Food Microbiol* 2016 Jan 18, 217 pp 195–99.

111. Ponsonby, A. L. et al., 'Exposure to infant siblings during early life and risk of multiple sclerosis', *JAMA* 293, no 4, Jan 2005, pp 463–69.

112. Van der Mei, I. A. et al., 'Past exposure to sun, skin phenotype, and risk of multiple sclerosis: case-control study', *BMJ* (clinical research ed.) vol 327, no 7410, Aug 2003, p 316.

113. Ascherio, A., 'Environmental factors in multiple sclerosis', *Expert review of neurotherapeutics*, vol 13, no 12, suppl. Dec. 2013, pp 3–9.

114. Kfoczynska, M. et al., 'The role of Vitamin D in multiple sclerosis', *Polstepy Hig Med Dosw* (online) 8 April 2015, 69 pp 440–48.

115. Ascherio, A., 'Environmental factors in multiple sclerosis', *Expert Rev Neuroth* 2013 Dec 13 (suppl 12) pp 3–9.

116. Groves, N. J. et al., 'Vitamin D as a neurosteroid affecting the developing and adult brain', *Annu Rev Nutr* 2014, 34, pp 117–41.

117. Durk, M. R. et al., '1α-25-Dihydroxyvitamin D3 reduces cerebral amyloid-β accumulation and improves cognition in mouse models of Alzheimer's disease', *J Neurosci*, 21 May 2014, 34(21) 7091–101.

118. Shaygannejad, V. et al., 'What is the real Fate of Vitamin D in Multiple Sclerosis?', *Int J Prev Med*, 4 May 2013, suppl 2 pp 159–64.

119. FDA (U.S. Food and Drug Administration), http://usatoday30.usatoday.com/news/health/2008-06-12-dental-fillings_N.htm.

120. Craelius, S., 'Comparative epidemiology of multiple sclerosis and dental caries', *J Epidemiol Comm Health*, 32 1978(5) pp 155–65.

121. Anglen, J. et al., 'Occupational mercury exposure in association with prevalence of multiple sclerosis and tremor among US dentists', *J Am Dent Assoc*, 2015 Sept, 146(9) pp 659–68.e.1.

122. Svare, C. et al., 'The effects of dental amalgams on mercury levels in expired air', *J Dent Res*, 60 1081 pp 1668–71.

123. McGrother, C. W. et al., 'Multiple sclerosis, dental caries and fillings: a case-control study', *Br Dent J*, 11 Sept 1999, 187(5) pp 261–64.

124. Napier, M. D. et al., 'Heavy metals, organic solvents, and multiple sclerosis: An exploratory look at gen-environment interactions', *Arch Environ Occup Health*, 19 Aug 2014, 19 pp 1–9.

125. Attar, A. M. et al., 'Serum mercury level and multiple sclerosis', *Biol Trace Elem Res.*, May 2012, 146(2) pp 150–53.

126. Ingalls, Th., 'Epidemiology, etiology, and prevention of multiple sclerosis: hypothesis and fact', *Am J Forensic Med Pathol*, 4 Mar 1983, (1) pp 55–61.

127. Siblerud, R. L. et al., 'Evidence that mercury from silver dental fillings may be an etiological factor

in multiple sclerosis', *Sci Total Environ*, 15 Mar 1994,142(3) pp 191–205.
128. Affelska, J.A., 'The toxic effect of mercury in occupational exposure', *Med Pr*, 1999, 50(4) pp 305–14.
129. Prochazkova, J. et al., 'The beneficial effect of amalgam replacement on health in patients with autoimmunity', *Neurol Endocriniol Lett.*, June 2004, 25(3) pp 2011–18.
130. Huggins, H.A. et al., 'Cerebrospinal fluid protein changes in multiple sclerosis after dental amalgam removal', *Altern Med Rev*, 3 Aug 1998, (4) pp 295–300.
131. Evers, J., *Warum Evers-Diät? Die Ernährung des Gesunden und Kranken*, Haug Verlag Stuttgart, 12th edition 1992, ISBN: 3-7760-1071-1.
132. Farez, M.F. et al., 'Sodium intake is associated with increased activity in multiple sclerosis', *J Neurol Neurosurch Psychiatry*, Jan 2015, 86(1) pp 26–31.
133. Krementsov, D.N. et al., 'Exacerbation of autoimmune neuroinflammation by dietary sodium is genetically controlled and sex specific', *FASEB J*, Aug 2015, 29(8) pp 3446–57.
134. Hernandez, A.L. et al., 'Sodium chloride inhibits the suppressive function of FOXP3 + regulatory T cells', *J Clin Invest*, 2 Nov 2015, 125(11) pp 4212–22.
135. Hewson, D.C. et al., 'Food intake in multiplesclerosis', *Hum Nutr Appl Nutr*, Oct 1984, 38(5) pp 355–67.
136. Ben-Shlomo, Y. et al., 'Dietary fat in the epidemiology of multiple sclerosis: has the situation been adequately assessed?', *Neuroepidemiology*, 1992, 11(4–6) pp 214–25.
137. Schwarz, S., 'Multiple sclerosis and nutrition', abstract supplement, *Progress in MS Research*, Oct. 2015, Melbourne, online: http://msj.sagepub.com/ content/11/1/24.abstract.
138. Payne, A., 'Nutrition and diet in the clinical management of multiple sclerosis', *J Hum Nutr Diet* 2001 Oct 14(5) pp 349–57.
139. Di Biase, A. et al., 'Eicosapentaenoic acid pretreatment reduces biochemical changes induced in total brain and myelin of weaning Wistar rats by cuprizone feeding', *Prostaglandins Leukot Essent Fatty Acids*, 2014 Apr 90(4) pp 99–104.
140. Farinotti, M. et al., 'Dietary intervention for multiple sclerosis', *Cochraine Database Syst Rev.* 2012 Dec 12,12CD004192, doi:10.1002/14651858, CD004192.pub3.
141. McDougall, J.A., 'Treating Multiple Sclerosis with Diet: Fact or Fraud?', Physicians Committee online (http://www.pcrm.org/health/health-topics/treating-multiples-sclerosis-with-diet-fact-or).
142. Hoare, S. et al., 'Higher intake of omega-3 polyunsaturated fatty acids is associated with a decreased risk of a first clinical diagnosis of central nervous system demyelinisation: Results from the Ausimmune Study', *Mult Scler* 2015 Sep 11, Pii:1352458515604380. (Epub ahead of print).
143. Weinstock-Guttmann, B. et al., 'Low fat dietary intervention with omega-3 fatty acid supplementation in multiple sclerosis patients', *Prostaglandins Leukot Essent Fatty Acids*, 2005 Nov 73(5) pp 397–404.
144. Mauriz, E. et al., 'Effects of low fat diet with anti-oxidant supplementation on biochemical markers of multiple sclerosis long-term card residents', *Nutr Hosp* 2013 Nov 1, 28(6) pp 2229–35.
145. Davis, W. et al., 'The fat mass and obesity-associated FTO rs9939609 polymorphism is associated with elevated homocysteine levels in patients with multiple sclerosis screened for vascular risk factors', *Metab Brain Dis.* 2014 June, 29(2) pp 409–19.
146. Saka, M. et al., 'Nutritional status and anthropometric measurements of patients with multiple sclerosis', *Saudi Med J* 2012 Feb 33(2) pp 160–66.
147. Sepcic, J. et al., 'Nutritional factors and multiple sclerosis in Gorski Kotar, Croatia', *Neuroepidemiology* 1993 12(4) pp 234–40.
148. Tola, M.R. et al., 'Dietary habits and multiple sclerosis: A retrospective study in Ferrara, Italy', *Acta Neurol* (Naples) 1994 Aug 16(4) pp 189–97.
149. Geeta, S.M. et al., 'Dietary patterns in clinical subtypes of multiple sclerosis: an exploratory study', *Nutrition Journal* 2009 8:36 doi:10.1186/1475 – 2891-8-36.
150. Taylor, K.L. et al., 'Lifestyle factors, demographics and medications associated with depression risk in an international sample of people with multiple sclerosis', *BMC Psychiatry* 2014 Dec 3,14 pp 327.
151. Riccio, P. et al., 'Nutrition Facts and Multiple Sclerosis', *ASN neuro* 2015 2015 Feb 7(1), published online, doi:10.1177/1759091414568185.

152 Hadgkiss, E.J. et al., 'The association of diet with quality of life, disability, and relapse rate in an international sample of people with multiple sclerosis', *Nutr Neurosci* 2015 Apr, 18(3) pp 125–36.

153 Riccio, P. et al., 'May diet and dietary supplements improve the wellness of multiple sclerosis patients? An approach', *Autoimmune Dis* 2010; 2010 249842 published online 2011 Feb 24, doi:10.4061/2010/249842.

154 Soodeh, R.J. et al., 'Dietary patterns and risk of multiple sclerosis', *Iran J Neurol* 2012.11(2) pp 47–53.

155 Galland, L., 'The gut microbiome and the brain', *J Md Food* 2014 Dec 17(12) pp 1261–72.

156 Mielcarz, D.W. et al., 'The gut microbiome in multiple sclerosis', *Curr Treat Opinions Neurol* 2015, Apr 17(4) p 344.

157 Riccio, P., 'The molecular basis of nutritional intervention in multiple sclerosis: a narrative review', *Complement Ther Med* 2011 Aug 19(4) pp 228–37.

158 Erentheil, O.F. et al., 'The role of food allergy in multiple sclerosis', *Trans Am Assoc* 1951, 56 pp 234–6.

159 Jonez, H.D., 'The allergic aspects of multiple sclerosis', *Calif Med* 1953 Nov, 79(5) pp 376–80.

160 Pressemitteilung Universität Freiburg, 'Darmbakterien sorgen für gesundes Gehirn', 1 June 2015 (https://www.uniklinik-freiburg.de).

161 Sanoobar, M. et al., 'Coenzym Q10 supplementation ameliorates inflammatory markers in patients with multiple sclerosis: a double-blind, placebo-controlled randomized clinical trial', *Nutr Neurosci* 2015 May 18(4) pp 169–76.

162 Zahednasab, H., 'Coenzyme Q10 supplementation and multiple sclerosis', *Nutr Neurosci* 2015. May 18(4) p 192.

163 Khalili, M. et al., 'Does lipoic acid consumption affect the cytokine profile in multiple sclerosis patients: a double-blind, placebo-controlled randomized clinical trial', *Neuroimmunomodulation* 2014, 21(6) pp 291–96.

164 Harbige, L.S. et al., 'Polyunsaturated fatty acids in the pathogenesis and treatment of multiple sclerosis', *Br J Nutr* 2007 Oct 98 suppl 1 pp 46–53.

165 Millar, J.H. et al., 'Double-blind trial of linoleate supplementation of the diet in multiple sclerosis', *Br Med J* 1973 Mar 31, 1(5856) pp 765–8.

166 Bates, D. et al., 'Polyunsaturated fatty acids in treatment of acute remitting multiple sclerosis', *Br Med J* 1978 Nov 18, 2(6149) pp 1390–1.

167 Seidel, D., 'Polyunsaturated (essential) fatty acids and their importance in pathogenesis diagnosis and therapy of multiple sclerosis', *Fortschr Neurol Psychiatr* 1982 June, 50(6) pp 173–89.

168 Glabinski, A. et al., 'Increased generation of superoxide radicals in the blood of MS patients', *Acta Neur Scand* 1993 Sept, 88(3) pp 174–77.

169 Syburra, C. et al., 'Oxydative stress in patients with multiple sclerosis', *Ukr Biokhim Zh* 1999 May–June, 71(3) pp 112–15.

170 Polachini, C.R. et al., 'Evolution of delta-aminolaevulinic dehydratase activity, oxydative stress biomarkers, and vitamin D levels in patients with multiple sclerosis', *Neurotox Res* 2015 Dec 21. PMID 26690779.

171 Socha, G. et al., 'Dietary habits and selenium, glutathione peroxidase and total antioxidant status in the serum of patients with relapsing-remitting multiple sclerosis', *Nutr J* 2014 June 18, 13 p 62.

172 Liu, J. et al., 'Microglial Hv1 proton channel promotes cuprizone-induced demyelination through oxidative dammage', *J Neurochem* 2015 Oct 135(2) pp 347–56.

173 Vakilzadeh, G. et al., 'The effect of melatonin on behavioral, molecular, and histopathological changes in curpizone model of demyelination', *Mol Neurobiol* 2015 Aug 27. PMID 26310973.

174 Jennwitheesuk, A. et al., 'Melatonin regulates aging and neurodegeneration through energy metabolism, epigenetics, autophagy and circadian rhythm pathways', *J Mol Sci* 2014 Sept 22, 15(9) pp 16848–84.

175 Yadav, S.K. et al., 'Advances in the immunopathogenesis of multiple sclerosis', *Curr Opin Neurol* 2015 June 28(3) pp 206–19.

176 Vijayshree, Y. et al., 'Effects of a low-fat plant-based diet in multiple sclerosis (MS): results of a one-year-long randomized controlled (RC) study', *Neurology* 8 April 2014 vol 82 no 10 supplement P6.152.

177 McCarty, M.F., 'Upregulation of lymphocyte apoptosis as a strategy for preventing and treat-

ing autoimmune disorders: a role for whole-food vegan diets, fish oil and dopamine agonists', *Medical Hypotheses*, 2001, Aug 57(2) pp 258–75.

178. Vakusic, S. et al., 'Pregnancy and multiple sclerosis (the PRIMS study): clinical predictors of post-partum relapse', *Brain* vol 127, pt 6, June 2004, pp 1353–1360.

179. Rolak, L.A. et al., 'The differential diagnosis of multiple sclerosis', *The Neurologist* vol. 13 no 2 March 2007 pp 57–72.

180. Weinshenker, B.G. et al., 'A randomized trial of plasma exchange in acute central nervous system inflammatory demyelinating disease', *Ann of Neurol* vol 46 (6) Dec 1999 pp 878–86.

181. Sutton, D.M. et al., 'Complications of plasma exchange', *Transfusion*. 29 (2) Feb 1989, pp 124–27.

182. De Jong et al., 'Confusing Cochrane reviews on treatment in multiple sclerosis', *Lancet neurol* 4(6) Jun 2005 pp 330–31.

183. Europäische Gesundheitsbehörde EPAR, 'Zusammenfassung für die Öffentlichkeit' (http://www.ema.europa.eu/docs/de) February 2014.

184. Pöllmann et al., *Therapie von Schmerzen bei MS – eine Übersicht mit evidenzbasierten Therapieempfehlungen*, Fortschr Neurologie Psychiatrie vol 73(5) May 2005 pp 268–85.

185. Blanco et al., 'Autologous haemopatopoietic-stem-cell transplantation for multiple sclerosis', *Lancet neurology* vol 4 (1) Jan 2005 pp 54–63.

186. Spillantini, M.G. et al., 'Alpha synuclein in Lewi bodies', *Nature* vol 388 no 665 Aug 1997 pp 839–840.

187. Singleton, A.B. et al., '*Alpha-synuclein locus triplication causes Parkinson's disease*', *Science* vol 302 no 5646 Oct 2003 p 841.

188. Fuchs, J. et al., 'Genetic variability in the SNCA-gene influences alpha-synuclein levels in the blood and brain', *FASEB journal* vol 22 no 5 May 2008 pp 1327–1334.

189. Chin-Chan, M. et al., 'Environmental polluants as risk factors for neurodegenerative disorders such as Alzheimer and Parkinson's disease', *Front Cel Neurosci* 2015, Apr 10, 9 p 124. PMID: 25914525.

190. Lin, C.Y. et al., 'Dose-response relationship between cumulative mercury exposure index and specific uptake ratio in the striatum on Tc-99m TRODAT SPECT', *Clin Nucl Med* 2011 Aug, 36(8) pp 689–93.

191. Dantzig, P.L., 'Parkinson's disease, macular degeneration and cutaneous signs of mercury toxicity', *J Occup Environ Med* 2006 July 48(7) p 656.

192. Carpenter, D.O., 'Effects of metals on the nervous system of humans and animals', *Int J Occup Med Environ Health* 2001, 14(3) pp 209–18.

193. Finkelstein, Y. et al., 'The enigma of Parkinsonism in chronic borderline mercury intoxication, resolved by challenge with penicillamine', *Neurotoxicology* spring 1996, 17(1) pp 219–6.

194. Reinhardt, J.W., 'Side effects: mercury contribution in body burden from dental amalgam', *Adv Dent Res* 1991 Sept 6 pp 110–13.

195. Ngim, C.H. et al., 'Epidemiologic study on the association between body burden mercury level and idiopathic Parkinson's disease', *Neuroepidemiology* 1989, 8(3) pp 128–41.

196. Ngim, C.H. et al., 'Epidemiologic study on the association between body burden mercury level and idiopathic Parkinson's disease', *Neuroepidemiology* 1989, 8(3) pp 128–41.

197. Pham, A.N. et al., 'Cu(II)-catalized oxidation of dopamine in aqueous solutions: mechanism and kinetics', *J Inorg Biochem* 2014 Aug vol 137 pp 74–84.

198. Davies, K.M. et al., 'Copper pathology in vulnerable brain regions in Parkinson's disease', *Neurobiol Aging* 2014 April, 35(4) pp 858–66.

199. Double, K.L., 'Neuronal vulnerability in Parkinson's disease', *Parkinsonism Relat Disord* 2012 Jan 18 suppl 1 pp 52–4.

200. Montes, S. et al., 'Copper and copper proteins in Parkinson's disease', *Oxid Med Cell Longev* 2014 pp 147–251.

201. Gorell, J.M. et al., 'Occupational metal exposures and the risk of Parkinson's disease', *Neuroepidemiology* 1999, 18(6) pp 303–6.

202. Rybicke, B.A. et al., 'Parkinson's disease mortality and the industrial use of heavy metals in Michigan', *Mov Disord*. 1993, 8(1) pp 87–92.

203. Zecca, L. et al., 'New melanic pigments in the human brain that accumulate in aging and block environmental toxic metals', *Proc Natl Acad Sci USA* 2008 Nov 11, 105(45) pp 17567–72.

204. Dusek, P. et al., 'The neurotoxicity of iron, copper and manganese in Parkinson's and Wilson's diseases,' *J Trace Elem Med Biol*. 2015, 31 pp 193–203.

205. Fukushima, T et al., 'Relationship between blood levels of heavy metals and Parkinson's disease in China', *Neuroepidemiology* 2010, 34(1) pp 18–24.
206. Pearce, R. K. et al., 'Alterations in the distribution of glutathione in the substantia nigra in Parkinson's disease', *J Neural Transm* (Vienna) 1997, 104(6–7) pp 661–77.
207. Caudle, S. M., 'Occupational exposures and Parkinsonism', *Handb Clin Neurol* 2015, 131 pp 225–39.
208. Wan, N. et al., 'Parkinson's disease and pesticide exposure: new findings from a comprehensive study in Nebraska', *J Rural Health* 2015 Oct 30.doi:10.1111/jrh.12154 (e-pub ahead of print).
209. Narayan, S. et al., 'Genetic variability in ABCB1, occupational pesticide exposure, and Parkinson's disease', *Environ Res* 2015 Nov, 143(Pt A) pp 98–106.
210. James, K.A. et al., 'Groundwater pesticide levels and the associations with Parkinson disease', *Int J Toxicol* 2015 May–June 34(3) pp 266–73.
211. Searles, N.S. et al., 'Blood α-synuclein levels in agricultural pesticide handlers in central Washington State', *Environ Re.* 2015 Jan 136 pp 75–81.
212. Van der Mark, M. et al., 'Occupational exposure to pesticides and endotoxin and Parkinson's disease in the Netherlands', *Occup Environ Med* 2014 Nov, 71(11) pp 757–64.
213. Baltazar, M.T. et al., 'Pesticides exposure as etiological factors of Parkinson's disease and other neurodegenerative disease – a mechanistic approach', *Toxicol Lett* 2014 Oct 15, 230(2) pp 85–103.
214. Wang, A. et al., 'The association between ambient exposure to organophosphates and Parkinson's disease risk', *Occup Env Med* 2014 April, 71(4) pp 275–81.
215. Aboud, A.A. et al., 'PARK2 patient neuroprogenitors show increased mitochondrial sensitivity to copper', *Neurobiol Dis* 2015 Jan, 73 pp 204–12.
216. Ohlson, C.G. et al., 'Parkinson's disease and occupational exposure to organic solvents, agricultural chemicals and mercury – a case-referent study', *Scand J Work Environ Health* 1981 Dec, 7(4) pp 252–6.
217. Goldman, S.M., 'Environmental toxins and Parkinson's disease', *Annu Rev Pharmavol Toxicol* 2014, 54 pp 141–64.
218. Taetzsch, T. et al., 'Pesticides, microglial NOX2, and Parkinson's disease', *J Biochem Mol Toxicol* 2013 Feb, 27(2) pp 137–49.
219. Singh, N.K. et al., 'Gene-gene and gene-environment interaction on the risk of Parkinson's disease', *Curr Aging Sci* 2014, 7(2) pp 101–9.
220. Liu, X. et al., 'Pesticide-induced gene mutations and Parkinson's disease risk: a meta-analysis', *Genet Test Mol Biomarkers* 2013 Nov, 17(11) pp 826–32.
221. Dardiotis, E. et al., 'The interplay between environmental and genetic factors in Parkinson's disease susceptibility: the evidence for pesticides', *Toxicology* 2013 May 10, 307 pp 17–23.
222. *Sci Signal*, 'A Trojan horse for Parkinson's disease', *Sci Signal* 2010 April 6, 3 p 116.
223. Ratner, M.H. et al., 'Younger age at onset of sporadic Parkinson's disease among subjects occupationally exposed to metals and pesticides', *Interdiscip Toxicol* 2014 Sept 7(3) pp 123–33.
224. Yong-Kee, C.J. et al., 'Mitochondrial dysfunction precedes other sub-cellular abnormalities in an in vitro model linked with cell death in Parkinson's disease'. University of Toronto, 2013.
225. Choi, W.S. et al., 'Loss of mitochondrial complex I activity potentiates dopamine neuron death induced by microtubule dysfunction in a Parkinson's disease model', *J Cell Biol* 2011 March 7, 192(5) pp 873–82.
226. Chin-Chan, M. et al., 'Environmental pollutants as risk factors for neurodegenerative disorders: Alzheimer and Parkinson diseases', *Front. Cel Neurosci* 2015 April 10, 9 p 124.
227. Blesa, J. et al., 'Oxidative stress and Parkinson's disease', *Front Neuroanat* 2015 July 8, 9 p 91.
228. Sanders, L.H. et al., 'Oxidative damage to macromolecules in human Parkinson's disease and the rotenone model', *Free Radic Biol Med* 2013 Sept, 62 pp 110–120.
229. Ward, J., 'Free radicals, antioxidants and preventive geriatrics', *Aust Fam Physician* 1994 July, 23(7) pp 1297–1301 and 1305.
230. Khan, M.S. et al., 'Targeting Parkinson's-tyrosine hydroxylase and oxidative stress as points of interventions', *CNS Neurol disord Drug Targets* 2012 June 1, 11(4) pp 369–80.
231. Kones, R., 'Parkinson's disease: mitochondrial molecular pathology, inflammation, statins, and

therapeutic neuroprotective nutrition', *Nutr Clin Pracdt* 2010 Aug, 25 pp 371–89.

232 Kim, T., 'A Guide to Neurotoxic Animal Models of Parkinson's Disease', *Cold Spring Harbor Perspectives in Medicine*, vol 1 no 1 Sept 2011, a009316.

233 J. et al., 'Targeted toxicans to dopaminergic neuronal cell death', *Methods Mol Biol* 2015, 1254 pp 239–52.

234 Checkosay, H. et al., 'Epidemiologic approaches to the study of Parkinson's disease etiology', *Epidemiology* 1999 May, 10(3) pp 327–36.

235 Barbeau, A. et al., 'Environmental and genetic factors in the etiology of Parkinson's disease', *Advances in Neurology* vol 45, 1987, pp 299–306.

236 Francisco, P.M. et al., 'Environmental toxins trigger PD-like progression via increased alpha-synuclein release from enteric neurons in mice', *Scientific Reports* 2, no 898, 2012.

237 Focus online: 'Pestizide in der Landwirtschaft: Parkinson gilt in Frankreich als Berufskrankheit', http://www.focus.de/gesundheit/ratgeber/ gehirn/ news/pestizide-in-der-landwirtschaft-frankreich-billigt-parkinson-als-berufskrankheit_ aid_751332.html, Focus online, 11 May 2012, viewed on 15 Sept 2015.

238 Hu, Y. et al., 'A Trojan horse for Parkinson's disease', *Sci Signal* 2010 April 6, 3(116) pe 13. PMID 20371768.

239 Caudl, W.M. et al., 'Industrial toxins and Parkinson's disease', *Neurotoxicology* 2012 March, 33(2) pp 178–88.

240 Inamdar, A.A. et al., 'Fungal-derived semiochemical 1-octen-3-ol disrupts dopamine packaging and causes neurodegeneration', *Proceedings of the National Academy of Sciences*, doi:10.1973/pnas 1318830110, https://dx.doi.org/10.1073%2Fn-pas.1318830110.

241 Xu, Q. et al., 'Diabetes and risk of Parkinson's disease', *Diabetes Care* 2011 April, 34(4) 910–5.

242 Chen, H. et al., 'Smoking duration, intensity and risk of Parkinson's disease', *Neurology* 2010 Mar 16, 74(11) pp 878–84.

243 Ma, L. et al., 'Dietary factors and smoking as risk factors for PD in a rural population in China: a nested case-control study', *Acta Neurol Scand* 2006 April, 113(4) pp 278–81.

244 Wirdefeldt, K. et al., 'Epidemiology and etiology of Parkinson's disease: a review of the evidence', *Eur J Epidemiol* 2011 June, 26 suppl 1, pp 1–85.

245 Schütz, J. et al., 'Risks for central nervous system disease among mobile phone subscribers: a Danish retrospective cohort study', *PLOS One* 2009, 4(2) e4389. doi:10.1371/journal.pone. 0004389 (e-pub 5 Feb 2009).

246 Zhang, D. et al., 'Alcohol intake and risk of Parkinson's disease: a meta-analysis of observational studies', *Mov Disord* 2014 May, 29(6) pp 819–22.

247 Eriksson, A.K. et al., 'Alcohol use disorders and risk of Parkinson's disease: findings from a Swedish national cohort study 1972–2008', *BMC Neurol* 2013 Dec 5, pp 13–190.

248 Palacios, N. et al., 'Alcohol risk of Parkinson's disease in a large prospective cohort of men and women', *Mov Disord* 2012 July, 27(9) pp 960–7.

249 Dong, J. et al., 'Dietary fat intake and Parkinson's disease', *Mov Disord* 2014 Nov, 29(13) pp 1623–30.

250 Ross, G.W. et al., 'Association of coffee and caffeine intake with the risk of Parkinson's disease', *HAMA* 2000 May 24–31, 283(20) pp 2674–9.

251 Tanaka, K. et al., 'Intake of Japanese and Chinese teas reduces risk of Parkinson's disease', *Parkinsonism Relat Disord* 2011 July,17(6) pp 446–50.

252 Agim, Z.S. et al., 'Dietary factors in the etiology of Parkinson's disease', *Biomed Res Int* 2015 pp 672–838.

253 Collins, M.A., 'Alkaloids, alcohol and Parkinson's disease', *Parkinsonism Related Disord* 2002 Sept, 8(6) pp 417–22.

254 Schlesinger, I. et al., 'Uric acid in Parkinson's disease', *Mov Disord* 2008 Sept 15, 23(12) pp 1653–7; Ellwanger, J.H. et al., 'Selenium reduces bradykinesis and DNA-damage in a rat model of Parkinson's disease', *Nutrition* 2015 Feb, 31(2) pp 359–65.

255 Zhu, B.T, 'CNS dopamine oxidation and catechol-O-methyltransferase: importance in the etiology, pharmacotherapy, and dietary prevention of Parkinson's disease', *Int J Mol Med* 2004 March, 13(3) pp 343–53.

256 Duan, W. et al., 'Dietary Folate deficiency and elevated homocysteine levels endanger dopaminergic neurons, in models of Parkinson's disease', *J Neurochem* 2002 Jan, 80 pp 101–10.

257 Murakami, K. et al., 'Dietary intake of folate, vitamin B6, vitamin B12 and riboflavin and risk of Parkinson's disease: a case-control study in Japan', *Br J Nutr* 2010 Sept,104(5) pp 757–64.

258 Spinelli, K.J., 'Curcumin Treatment Improves Motor Behavior in α-Synuclein Transgenic Mice', *PLOS One* 2015 June 2, 10(6), eO128510, PMID 26035833, PMCID PMC4452784.

259 Siddique, Y.H. et al., 'Effects of curcumin on life span, activity pattern, oxidative stress, and apoptosis in brains of transgenic Drosophila model of Parkinson's disease', *Biomed Res int*. 2014, 2014:606928 (e-pub April 17). PMID 24860828.

260 Wang, L. et al., 'Vitamin D from different sources is inversely associated with Parkinson's disease', *Mov Disord* 2015 April, 30(4) pp 560–6.

261 Newmark, H.L. et al., 'Vitamin D and Parkinson's disease – a hypothesis', *Mov Disord* 2007 March 15, 22(4) pp 461–8.

262 Bousquet, M. et al., 'Impact of ω-3 fatty acids in Parkinson's disease', *Ageing Res Rev* 2011 Sept, 10(4) pp 453–63.

263 Knoes, R., 'Parkinson's disease: mitochondrial molecular pathology, inflammation, statins, and therapeutic neuroprotective nutrition', *Nutr Clin Pract* 2010 Aug, 25(4) pp 371–89.

264 De Lau, L.M. et al., 'Dietary fatty acids and the risk of Parkinson disease: the Rotterdam study', *Neurology* 2005 June 28, 64(12) pp 2040–5.

265 Chen, H. et al., 'Diet and Parkinson's disease: a potential role of dairy products in men', *Ann Neuro* 2002 Dec, 52(6) pp 793–801.

266 Grant, W.B., 'The role of milk protein in increasing risk of Parkinson's disease', *Eur J Epidemiol* 2013 April, 28(4) p 357.

267 Powers, K.M. et al., 'Parkinson's disease risks associated with dietary iron, manganes, and other nutrient intakes', *Neurology* 2003 June 10, 60(11) pp 1761–6.

268 Griffioen, K.J. et al., 'Dietary energy intake modifies brainstem autonomic dysfunction caused by mutant α-Synuclein', *Neurobiol Aging* 2013 March, 34(3) pp 928–35.

269 Johnson, C.C. et al., 'Adult nutrient intake as a risk factor for Parkinson's disease', *Int J Epidemol* 1999 Dec, 28(6) pp 1102–9.

270 Logroscino, G. et al., 'Dietary iron, animal fats, and risk of Parkinson's disease', *Mov Disord* 1998, 13 suppl 1 pp 13–6.

271 Morris, J.K. et al., 'Insulin resistance impairs nigrostriatal dopamine function', *Exp Neurol* 2011 Sept, 23(1) pp 171–80.

272 Duarte, J. et al., 'Efficacy of the proteic redistribution diet (PRD) in the antiparkinsonian effect of L-dopa', *Neurologie* 1993 Oct, 8(8) pp 248–51.

273 Karstaedt, P. et al., 'Protein redistribution diet remains effective in patients with fluctuating parkinsonism', *Arch Neurol* 1992 Feb, 49(2) pp 149–51.

274 Croxson, S. et al., 'Dietary modification of Parkinson's disease', *Eur J Clin Nutr* 1991 May, 45(5) pp 263–6.

275 Astarloa, R. et al., 'Clinical and pharmacokinetic effects of a diet rich in insoluble fiber on Parkinson's disease', *Clin Neuropharmacol* 1992 Oct 15(5) pp 375–80.

276 Harv Health Lett Jun 2012, 'Flavonoids may help protect against Parkinson's disease', Harv Health Lett 2012 June, 37(8) p 8 (no author cited).

277 Miyake, Y. et al., 'Dietary intake of antioxidant vitamins and risk of Parkinson's disease: a case-control study in Japan', *Eur J Neurol* 2011 Jan, 18(1) pp 106–13.

278 Etminan, M. et al., 'Intake of vitamin E, vitamin C, and carotenoids and risk of Parkinson's disease: a meta-analysis', *Lancet Neurol* 2005 June, 4(6) pp 362–5.

279 Ferraz, H.B. et al., 'Comments on the paper "High doses of riboflavin and the elimination of dietary red meat promote the recovery of some motor functions in Parkinson's disease patients"', *Braz J Med Biol Res* 2004 Sept, 37(9) pp 1297–9.

280 Coimbra, C.G. et al., 'High doses of riboflavin and the elimination of dietary red meat promote the recovery of some motor functions in Parkinson's disease patients', *Braz J Med Biol Res* 2003 Oct, 36(10) pp 1409–17.

281 Logroscino, C. et al., 'Dietary iron, animal fats, and risk of Parkinson's disease', *Mov Disord* 1998, 13 suppl 1 pp 13–6.

282 Rabey, J.M. et al., 'Broad bean (vicia faba) consumption and Parkinson's disease', *Adv Neurol* 1993, 60 pp 681–4.

283 Alkalay, R.N. et al., 'The association between Mediterranean diet adherence and Parkinson's disease', *Mov Disord* 2012 May, 27(6) pp 771–4.

284 Di Giovanni, G., 'A diet for dopaminergic neurons?', *J Neural Transm Suppl* 2009, (73) pp 317–31.

285 Albarracin, S.L. et al., 'Effects of natural antioxidants in neurodegenerative disease', *Nutr Neurosci* 2012 Jan, 15(1) pp 1–9.

286 Okubo, H. et al., 'Dietary patterns and risk of Parkinson's disease: a case-control study in Japan', *Eur J Neurol* 2012 May, 19(5) pp 681–8.

287 Di Matteo, V. et al., 'Intake of tomato-enriched diet protects from 6-hydroxydopamine-induced degeneration of rat nigral dopaminergic neurons', *J Neural Transm* suppl. 2009, (73) pp 333–41.

288 Zhu, B.T., 'CNS dopamine oxidation and catechol – methyltransferase: importance in the etiology, pharmacotherapy, and dietary prevention of Parkinson's disease', *Int J Mol Med* 2004 March, 13(3) pp 343–53.

289 Zhang, S.M. et al., 'Intakes of vitamins E and C, carotenoids, vitamin supplements and PD risk', *Neurology* 2002 Oct 22, 59(8) pp 1161–9.

290 Baroni, L. et al., 'Pilot dietary study with normo-proteic protein-redistributed plant-food diet and motor performance in patients with Parkinson's disease', *Nutr Neurosci* 2011 Jan, 14(1) pp 1–9.

291 McCarty, M.F., 'Does a vegan diet reduce risk for Parkinson's disease?', *Med Hypothesis* 2001 Sept, 57(3) pp 318–23.

292 'Leitlinie Parkinson-Syndrom der Deutschen Gesellschaft für Neurologie' (http://www.dgn.org/images/stories(dgn/leitlinien/parkinson_mit_Tabellen.pdf).

293 Freedman, M., 'Parkinson's disease', Cummings, J.L., ed. *Subcortical Dementia*, Oxford University Press, New York, 1990, pp 108–22.

294 Beatty, W.W. et al., 'Analyzing the subcortical dementia syndrome of Parkinson's disease using the RBANS', *Arch Clin Neuropsychol* 2003, 18(5) pp 509–20.

295 Ju, He Kang, 'Association of cerebrospinal fluid β-amyloid 1-42, T-tau, P-tau(8), and α-synuclein levels with clinical features of drug-naïve patients with early Parkinson's disease', *JAMA Neurology*, 2013 pp 1277–87, doi:10.1001(jamaneurol.2013.3861).

296 Nutt, J.G. et al., 'Interference of certain aminoacids with L-dopa at the blood-brain barrier', *New Engl Journal of Medicine* 310 p 483, 1984.

297 Pincus, J.H. et al., *Arch Neurol* 44 p 279, 1984.

298 Bumann, C. et al., 'Effect of subthalamic nucleus deep brain stimulation on driving in Parkinson's disease', *Neurology*, doi:10.1212//01.wnl.0000438223.17976.fb (https:///dx.doi.org/10.1212%2F01.wnl.0000438223.17876.fb).

299 Watzel, B., and Leitzmann, C., *Bioaktive Substanzen in Lebensmitteln*, Hippokrates-Verlag, Stuttgart, ISBN 3 7773-1115-4, 1995.

300 Becher, G.R. et al., 'Analysis of micronutrients in foods', in Moon, T.E., and Micozzi, M.S.(eds.), *Nutrition and cancer prevention: investigating the roles of micronutrients*, Decker, New York 1988, pp 103–58.

301 Hertog, M.G. et al., 'Optimization of a quantitative HPLC-determination of potentially anticarcinogenic flavonoids in vegetables and fruits', *J Agric Food Chem* 40 (1992), pp 1591–6.

302 Billings et al., 'Inhibition of radiation-induced transformation of CH3/10T1/2-cells by chymotrypsin-inhibitor 1 from potatoes', *Carcinogenesis* 8 (1987) pp 809–12.

303 Steinmetz, K.A. et al., 'Vegetables, fruit and cancer I and II', *Epidemiology, Cancer Causes Control* 2 (1991a) pp 325–57.

304 Steinmetz, K.A. und Potter J.D.: vegetables, fruit and cancer I and II, Epidemiology, Cancer-causes Control 2 (1991a) pp 325–57.

305 Birt T.F. et al: Chemoprevention by nutrient-components of vegetables and fruits. in: Alfin-Slater et al: Cancer and nutrition. Plenum Press, New York 1991, pp 221–60.

Index

α-synucleine	78, 82	arteriosclerosis	45, 49, 92
α-synuclein gene	78	astrocytes	18, 20, 35
β-cryptoxanthin	86	ataxia	42, 51, 52, 64
β-fibrils	32	autism	12, 40
δ-aminolevulinic acid dehydratase	61	autoimmune reaction	36
		avian tuberculosis	55
acetylcholine	17	axon	15, 39, 54, 63, 67
acid-base balance	18, 20		
ACTH	13	balo disease	28
action potential	17	basal ganglia	9, 11, 12, 17, 40, 43, 78, 83
acute motoric axonal neuropathy	28, 30		
adenohypophysis	13	basic regulation system	35
adenosine	47, 80	basic therapy	66
ADH	14, 18	B-cells	61
ADHS	45, 46	beer	46, 80
adrenalin	69	beta amyloids	31
agaricus muscaris	67, 68	beta folding-sheet structure	38
AIDS	65	bipolar disorder	12
akinesia	82, 84	bladder function impairment	67
alcohol	24, 46, 80	blood-brain barrier	18, 19, 20, 22, 23, 24, 25, 26, 35, 39, 40, 41, 46, 56, 65, 66, 68, 69, 79, 83
alcohol embryopathy (AE)	46		
allicin	88		
alpha liponic acid	85		
aluminium	78	blood capillaries	20, 32, 35
Alzheimer's dementia	32, 40, 41, 56, 81	blood pressure	12, 21, 32, 43, 44, 45, 47, 82
Alzheimer's disease	7, 8, 12, 25, 31, 32, 35, 38, 49, 50, 51, 79, 82, 86		
		blood pressure in the brain	21
		brad	82
amalgam and mercury vapours	57	bradykinesia	82
amalgam fillings	39, 57	bradyphrenia	78, 82
amantadine	83	brain liquid	83
amino acids	22, 23, 37, 83, 85, 87	brainstem	17, 84
		brain ventricles	23
amphetamines	44	breast milk	43
amyloidosis	32	bromide radical	38
amyotrophic lateral sclerosis (ALS)	38	bullying	50
anchovies	58, 79	butyrophenones	43
anthrozians	87		
anticholinergic substances	83	cadmium	43, 78
antigen-presenting cells in the brain	18	caffeine	47, 48, 80
antioxidative infusion treatment	85	calcium	16, 38, 39, 60
antioxidative substance	37, 61	campylobacter jejuni	30
apomorphine test	83	cancer	37, 41, 43, 45, 46, 47, 81, 86, 87, 88
aquaporin	14		
archipallium	12	cannabis	44, 67
arrhythmia	30, 42, 81	carboxylase inhibitor	83

carcinogens	87	cytochrome C	38
carotenoids	86	cytochrome P 450	37
catalase	37, 59, 61	cytokines	18, 22, 23, 29, 40, 47
cationic transport	22		
caudate nucleus	11	cytomegalovirus	30
cavities	19, 23, 57	cytoskeleton	35
CD-4 helper cells	61		
CD-8-suppressor cells	61	D2-receptors	40
cell membranes	15, 35, 37, 38, 39, 43, 61	dairy products	80, 97
		decarboxylase inhibitor	84
cell respiration	15, 38, 40	defecation	75
cerebellum	12, 17	delirium	46
cerebrum	10, 11, 12, 78	demyelinating diseases	28
chaos principle	34, 86	demyelination	30, 53
chaperone	38	dentric cells	7
chelation	57	depression	12, 42, 44, 45, 46, 49, 60, 67, 69
chemical respiratory chain	79		
chemokine	29	detoxification enzymes	37, 88
chinons	87	diabetes mellitus	55, 79
chlamydia	55	dialysis treatment	32
chloride radical	38	dichlorfluanid	43
chlorine	41	dietary treatment of	
chlorophyll	33	neurodegenerative diseases	86
cholera	22	disinfectant	41
cholesterol	15, 22, 27, 61	disseminated encephalomyelitis	
chorea minor	12	(ADEM)	28, 65
chrome	43	Disturbance of bladder emptying	64
cleaning agents	41, 79	DNA	33, 61, 86
coenzyme Q10	37, 60, 69, 85	DNA peroxidation	37
coffee	7, 47, 50, 60, 68, 80, 87	dopamine	11, 43, 44, 45, 78, 79, 81, 83, 84
cogwheel phenomenon	78, 82	dyskinesias	83
coherence	33, 86		
coherence principle of Prigogine	34	ECAM-1	60
collagenoses	65	effect of nutrition	33, 81
complement system	66	electromagnetic waves	26
comprehensive therapy	8	encephalopathy	42, 52
COMT-inhibitors	84	endorphins	45
concentration disorders	44	endothelial cells	20, 21, 23, 24, 41
connexin (CX32)	27	enteral immune system	8, 60, 89
contamination	58, 85	environmental toxins	7, 8, 68, 79
copper	39	epilepsy	53
corpora amygdalae	12	epiphysis	14, 61, 69
corpus callosum	10, 14	Epstein-Barr virus	30, 55, 61, 62
corpus mamillare	12	euphoria	45, 64
corpus striatum	9, 11, 84	executive cortex	10
corticobasal degeneration (CBD)	51	extrapyramidal motoric system	78
cramps	40, 44, 67, 73		
cyanosis	84	factor EGF	29

Faraday cage	26	heavy metals	8, 35, 43, 45, 48, 68, 80
fatty acids of animal-based food	80	hemiplegia	64
fava beans	81	heroin	45
fear	44, 45, 82	herpes viruses	55, 62
fish products, toxic metals	80	heterocyclic amines	80
flame retardants, neurotoxic substances	43	high-frequency radiation, pulsed	8
flavonoids	80, 86, 87	high in protein meals	83
flaxseed oil	60, 88	hippocampus	11, 12, 41, 43, 44
flu	63, 91	homocysteine	49, 59, 62, 80, 89
fluctuation (temporary deterioration)	83	homunculus	10
		hormone-producing glands	13
flu vaccination	30	hormone-releasing factor	13
foetal alcohol syndrome (FAS)	46	Huntington's disease	12, 17, 38
folic acid	22, 49, 60, 62, 68, 69, 80, 81, 85, 88	hydrocarbons, volatile organic	41
		hydrogen superoxide	18
food economy	35	hydrotherapy	71
fornix	12	hydroxide radical	37
FOX-P3+	59	hyperaesthesia	41
free radicals	38, 40, 61, 68, 80, 86, 88	hyperpathia	41
		hypokinesia	78
fresh vegetarian food	69	hypophysis	13
frontal lobes	10, 41, 43		
FSH	13	IgA-antibodies	8
funicular myelosis	28, 65	IgE	8
		IgG4	8, 62
GABA	17	immune competence	35, 89
galactocerebroside	27	immune defence	18, 20, 22
galacto-sulfatide	27	immune suppression	7
garlic	88, 103, 104, 109, 110, 112, 113, 114, 115, 117, 120, 121	immunological barrier	20
		inactivity atrophy	71
		inflammation	7, 8, 18, 29, 35, 41, 43, 46, 47, 49, 53, 55, 56, 59, 60, 61, 62, 65, 66, 68, 71, 88, 89, 90, 91
gene loci	55		
gene therapy	84		
glia cells	18		
glial scar	18		
globus pallidus	11, 12, 78	insomnia	40, 47, 51
GLUT-1	22	insulin	13, 22, 81
glutamate	17, 38	interferon	18, 23, 60, 66
glutathione	37, 49, 85	interleukins IL-1α	41
glutathione peroxidase	61	internuclear ophthalmoplegia	53
glutathione reductase	37	intestinal flora	8, 35, 60, 61, 69, 87, 89, 107
glycine	17		
growth hormone	13	intestinal mucosa	7, 60, 69, 87, 89
Guillain-Barré syndrome	30, 52	intestinal mucosa with putrefactive toxins	8
gyrus cinguli	12		
		irritability	45, 47
hair analyses and mercury content	57	isoelectrical focus	65
headache	42, 46, 47, 94	isoflavonoids	87

lab control recommendations for the attending physician during	89	meat, roasted	80
lack of appetite	40	Mediterranean diet	81
lack of movement	80, 84	medulla oblongata	12, 45
LASER	26, 33, 34, 86	melanocyte-stimulating hormone or melanotropin	14
LASER, amplification in our cells	33	melatonin	14, 61, 69
LDL cholesterol	61	MELISA	57
L-dopamine	84	memory	11, 12, 39, 41, 42, 43, 44, 45
L-Dopa test	83		
lead	40	meningea arachnoidea	19
lecithin	27	mental effects of Parkinson's syndrome	82
legal and prohibited drugs and neurodegenerative diseases	44	mental traumas	50
lemons	88, 99	menus for dietetic treatment	94
leucodystrophies	65	mesencephalon, midbrain	12
LEWY-bodies	78, 82	metabolic economy	35
LEWY-body dementia (LBD)	83	metal-based nanoparticles	79
Lhermitte sign	64	methylmercury	39, 40, 57
life energy	34, 69	MIBG-scintigraphy	83
lifestyle	7, 35, 37, 49, 50, 59, 68, 76, 86	microglia	20, 21, 23, 27, 29, 35, 56, 61, 79, 87
lignans, lignins	87		
limbic system	12, 41, 44	midbrain	12, 78
LINGO1	29	migraine	47, 92
linseed oil (flaxseed oil)	60, 62	Miller-Fisher syndrome	28
lipid peroxidation	37, 38, 43, 61	miscolonisation	60, 89
lipophilin	27	mitochondria	15, 37, 38, 40, 43, 60, 69, 79, 80
liquor cerebrospinalis	19, 57, 82		
loss of libido	82	MLCK, myosin light-chain kinase	24
LSD (lysergic acid diethylamide)	44	mobile phones	8, 26, 31
lutein	86	monoclonal antibody	66
luteinising hormone	13	Morbus Boeck	55
lycopene	86	Morbus Crohn	55
lymphocytes	8, 57, 59, 69	morphine	45
		morphogenetic fields	26
macroglia	20	motor cortex	10
macrophages	18, 21, 32, 35, 53, 61	motor neurons	51
		mould	39, 111
magnesium	16, 60	movement exercises	74
MAK	42	MSH	14
manganese	78, 81	mucosa barrier	8
MAO-inhibition	44	mucous, layer	8
mask-like face	82	mucuna pruriens	84
massages	74	multiple sclerosis	7, 8, 9, 18, 23, 29, 35, 36, 38, 50, 51, 53, 55, 57, 59, 60, 61, 62, 63, 64, 65, 66, 67, 68, 69, 71, 72, 73, 75, 76, 89
matrix	35, 69		
MCS, multiple chemical sensitivity	41		
MCT-1 and 2	22		
measles	65		
meat	7, 60, 68, 80		

multiple system atrophy (MSA)	51	neurotoxic medicines	43
muscarinic receptors	43	neurotransmitters	17, 18, 20, 38, 39, 43, 44, 45, 49, 78
myalgia	42		
mycobacterium	55	nickel	43
myelencephalon	12	nicotine	45
myelencephalon, afterbrain	12	nitrogen monoxide	18
myelin	7, 8, 15, 18, 27, 28, 29, 30, 35, 36, 37, 38, 40, 43, 46, 53, 54, 60, 61, 63, 65, 68	NMDA receptor	17, 43
		N-methyl-D-aspartate receptor (NMDA)	43
		non-ergo dopamine agonists	83
		noradrenaline	17, 44, 45, 49
myelin-associated glycoprotein (MAG)	27	NO-synthtase	38
		Notch-1-receptors	29
myelin oligodendrocyte glycoprotein (MOG)	27	NPSAH	61
		nucleus niger	9, 11
myeloproteine, basic (MBP)	65	nutrition and Parkinson's disease	80
		nystagmus	64
NADH (nicotinamide adenine dinucleotide hydrogen)	49	octenol	79
narcolepsy (forced sleeping during the day)	12	oedema	40, 84
		oligodendrocytes	18, 27, 29, 53, 65
		omega-3 fatty acids	59, 60, 62, 68, 80
necrosis factor 1 gene	55	opium	79
Neisseria meningitidis	22	opticus atrophy	64
nerve cells	8, 10, 11, 15, 16, 18, 31, 35, 38, 40, 43, 44, 46, 54, 73, 74, 78, 79, 80, 82, 86	order therapy	68
		organic solvents (VOC)	42
		organophosphates	42
		overheating treatment	74
neural therapy	67	oversensitivity of the skin to light	42
neurites	10, 15, 16, 47	oxytocin	18
neuroborreliose	65		
neurodegeneration	40, 42, 43, 88	pain	41, 42, 44, 45, 46, 64, 67, 82, 94
neurodegenerative diseases	7, 8, 9, 12, 22, 36, 37, 38, 39, 41, 42, 43, 48, 50, 51, 59, 75, 79, 80, 81, 83, 85, 87, 88, 89, 91, 107	pancreatitis	41, 46
		paralysis agitans	78
		paralysis, increasing	9
		Parkinsonism, atypical	82
		Parkinson's disease	7, 8, 9, 11, 12, 17, 38, 40, 43, 50, 51, 52, 78, 79, 80, 81, 82, 83, 85
neurohypophysis	14, 18		
neuroleptics	43, 84		
neuromyelitis optica	55		
neurons	10, 11, 13, 18, 26, 31, 35, 36, 46, 47, 54, 61, 69, 78, 79, 80, 83, 86	pericytes	21
		peripheral myeloprotein-22 (PMP-22)	27
		peripheral polyneuropathy	40
neuropathy, diabetic	38	personality, change of	42
neurosurgical treatment	84	pesticides	42, 43, 48, 79
neurotoxic harmful substances	43, 48	P-glycoprotein system	23
neurotoxicity	39, 42	phagocytosis	18, 32

141

pharmacological treatment	66, 83	refine textiles	40
phase II enzymes	87	remyelination	29, 30, 54, 64
phenol compounds	79	reserpine	43
phenoloxidase	87	respiratory arrest	44, 45
phenothiazines	43	restlessleg syndrome	82
phobias	12	retina	86, 87
phosphatidylethanolamine	27	retrobulbar neuritis	53, 64
photon	26, 33, 34, 83	rheumatic fever	12
photosynthesis	33, 86	riboflavin	80
phytochemicals	85	rickettsia	55
pill-turning tremor	78	rigor	78, 82, 84
plasmaphoresis	66	R.O.S.	37, 38, 40, 60, 61, 68
plexus chorioideus	19		
polybromated diphenyl ether (PBDE)	43	rubella	65
polyneuropathy	28, 41, 46	rutine	87
polyphenols	81, 87, 91		
polyradiculoneuropathy (SIDP)	30	S-Adenosyl methionine	49
pons	12	Salinon	41
posterior horn	13	salmon	58, 59, 78, 79
postural instability	82	salve face	82
potassium	16	scalar waves	26, 80
pre-frontal cortex	10	schizophrenia	44
pregnancy	40, 45, 46, 63, 79	Schwann cells	15, 27
primary effect	44	sea salt, mercury contamination	58
proantozianidine	80	secondary effects	44, 45, 48
problem-solving strategies	42	secondary plant substances (phytochemicals)	37, 62, 80, 86, 87
programmed cell death (apoptosis)	38		
progresses of MS	63	second main principle of thermodynamics	86
progressive supranuclear palsy (PSP)	51		
prolactine (PRL)	13	selenium	37, 61, 62, 80, 89
prostaglandins	23	sensitivity problems	64
protease inhibitors	87, 88	septum pellucidum	12
protein peroxidation	37	serotonin	17, 44, 45, 78
protein zero (P0, MPZ)	27	sexual function impairment	64
proteoglycans	35	sickbuilding syndrome	42
proteolipid protein (PLP/DM20)	27	silver	39
pseudo episode	63	sleep	7, 14, 49, 50, 61, 62, 69, 75
pulsed high-frequency radiation	26, 31, 73, 80		
pulse treatment	66	sleep, before midnight	7, 62, 69
putamen	78	sleeping-waking rhythm	11
pyrethroids	43	sleep, non-rem phases	69
		smoking	45
quercetin	87	social isolation	43
		sodium	16, 39, 41
radioactive contamination of food	58	somatotropin	13
Rauwolfia	43	speech disorders	44, 67
recipes	98	spinal cord	11, 12, 13, 15, 17, 19, 30, 37, 40, 46, 53, 69
red meat	81		
reduced sensitivity to touch	41		

142

Steele-Richardson-Olszewski syndrome	83	trigeminus neuralgia	64, 67
		tropical spastic paraparesis	65
STH	13	TSH	13, 89
streptococcus mutans	55	tumour necrosis factors 2	29
stress	7, 8, 12, 24, 35, 37, 38, 39, 40, 41, 42, 45, 47, 49, 50, 56, 58, 60, 61, 62, 68, 69, 79, 80, 81, 85, 86, 94	tumour necrosis factor α	18
		tuna	58, 78, 79
		twisted fibrils	31, 35, 79
		ubiquinone	37, 69, 85
		ultra-weak cell radiation	33
substantia nigra	11, 43, 78, 79, 80, 83	UVA radiation	37
subthalamic nucleus	12	varicella zoster viruses	65
sudden infant death	39	vascular dementia	49
suicidal tendencies	43	vasculitis	65
sunlight	26, 33	vasopressin	14
superoxyd dismutase	61	vegan diet	59, 62, 81
supporting measures for nursing	71	vegan raw food diet	93
supporting symptomatic treatment	67	vegetable L-dopamine	84
symptoms of Parkinson's disease	81	vegetable oils	7, 81, 88, 102
synapses	17, 20	vegetative nervous system	11, 17, 32, 35
syphilis	65	vesicular transport	22
		vision problems	42
table on the effects of foods onneurodegenerative diseases	90	visual problems	10, 11, 42, 45, 53, 54, 64, 66
		vitamin A	87
table on the general effect of raw food therapy	91	vitamin B6	49, 80, 85
table salt and multiple sclerosis	59	vitamin B12	46, 49, 80, 88
tauopathies	31	vitamin C	49, 61, 85, 87, 88, 95, 100
TAU proteins	31, 51, 82, 83	vitamin D	7, 49, 56, 60, 61, 62, 69, 72, 73, 80, 85, 88
temporal lobe	10		
terpens	88		
tetrabrombisphenol A (TBBA	43		
TGF-β	60	vitamin E	61, 62, 101
thalamus	11, 12, 13, 78		
thyroid	13	web-like cerebral membrane	19
tight junctions	20, 24	white substance of the brain	53
tin	39, 40, 41, 114	wholemeal wheat	87
T-lymphocytes	57	wine	46
TNF-α	23, 41	WLAN	8, 26, 73
toll-like receptors	29	wood-protection agents	42
tooth root abscesses	68		
toxic encephalopathy	41	xanthines	86
tractus corticospinalis	12		
transferrin	22	zeaxanthin	87
trembling	11, 78, 82, 84	zinc	46, 49, 78, 89
tremor	11, 40, 42, 46, 57, 78, 82, 84		
trichloroethylene	79		

CENTRE FOR SCIENTIFIC NATURAL MEDICINE

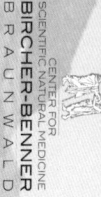

SCIENTIFIC NATURAL MEDICINE
CENTER FOR
BIRCHER-BENNER
BRAUNWALD

People come to the Bircher-Benner Medical Centre from a large number of countries in search of healing.

Here, you will be valued as a unique person, listened to and understood. Here, humanity and dignity are important and the medicine is a noble undertaking.

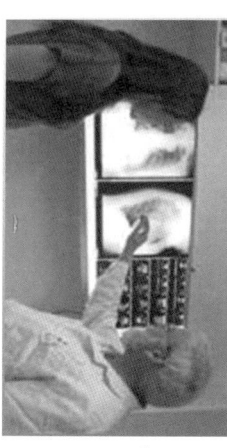

Centre for scientific natural medicine

Our fresh-vegetable diet will bring about a rapid change in your metabolism; natural regulative therapies take precedence where possible.

The atmosphere and the living tradition of the Bircher-Benner Centre, where novelty and modernity are combined with decades of experience, contribute to your healing.

The doctors and therapists will treat you personally and have all the facilities of a modern clinic at hand when needed.

The search for the true causes of diseases is central to our work, as is the inclusion of your self-curative powers in the process of healing.

Indications: *any internal diseases, migraine, tinnitus, neuralgia and other pain conditions, fibromyalgia, arthritis and arthrosis, collagenoses, liver, gallbladder and gastrointestinal diseases, metabolic diseases and diabetes, cardiovascular diseases, kidney and prostate diseases, women's diseases, allergies, skin diseases, convalescence, fatigue, depression and anxiety, menopausal, hormonal and weight problems.*

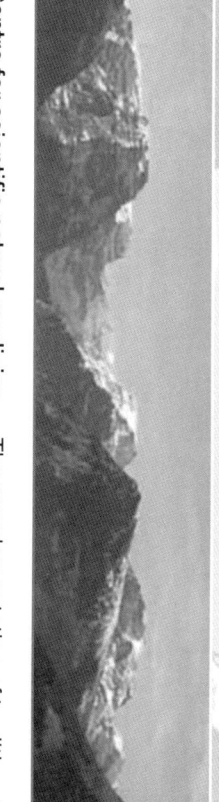

The supplementation of traditional medicine by the regulative diagnosis and therapy of natural healing often permits a cure where the usual therapies have failed.

In the Medical Centre, you can relax and recover, and will experience the deep regeneration of your healing powers.

CENTRE BIRCHER-BENNER
CH-8784 Braunwald
Phone: +41 (0)21 801 60 04
Fax: +41 (0)55 643 16 93
info@bircher-benner.com
www.bircher-benner.com